CLIMBING
THE
HEALTHCARE
MANAGEMENT
LADDER

WITHDRAWN
UTSA LIBRARIES

CLIMBING

THE
HEALTHCARE
MANAGEMENT
LADDER

Career Advice from the Top on How to Succeed

by
Jim Aldrich, M.H.S.A., M.B.A.

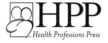

Baltimore • London • Sydney

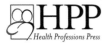

Health Professions Press, Inc.
Post Office Box 10624
Baltimore, Maryland 21285-0624

www.healthpropress.com

Copyright © 2013 by Health Professions Press, Inc.
All rights reserved.

Interior and cover designs by Mindy Dunn.
Typeset by Barton Matheson Willse & Worthington, Baltimore, Maryland.
Manufactured in the United States of America by Versa Press, East Peoria, Illinois.

This book is sold without warranties of any kind, express or implied, and the
publisher and author disclaim any liability, loss, or damage caused by the contents of
this book.

Library of Congress Cataloging-in-Publication Data

Aldrich, Jim.
  Climbing the healthcare management ladder : career advice from the top on how to
succeed / by Jim Aldrich.
      p. ; cm.
  Includes bibliographical references and index.
  ISBN 978-1-932529-97-5 (pbk.)
  I. Title.
  [DNLM: 1. Career Mobility. 2. Health Facility Administrators--organization
& administration. 3. Health Facility Administration. 4. Health Services
Administration. 5. Vocational Guidance. WX 155]
  RA971
  362.1068--dc23
                          2013002396

British Library Cataloguing in Publication data are available from the British Library.

**Library
University of Texas
at San Antonio**

Contents

About the Author

Jim Aldrich, M.H.S.A., M.B.A., is an emerging leader in the field of healthcare management. He is passionate about leadership and helping healthcare executives prepare for the challenges that lie ahead. A native of Michigan, Aldrich has more than 10 years of experience working in the field of healthcare.

Trained in Six Sigma and Lean Process improvement techniques, Aldrich served as Performance Improvement Specialist for St. Mary Mercy Hospital in Livonia, Michigan, and was responsible for coordinating emergency preparedness, contracting physicians for the Medical Staff Office, and managing nursing and performance improvement.

Following his own career path up the healthcare management ladder to what he hopes will become an executive position, Aldrich rose to his current position as Associate Director of Medical Staff Services in 2011 at St. Mary Mercy Hospital. He manages the daily operations of the Medical Staff Office and provides administrative oversight for physician contracting, credentialing, continuing medical education, and library services. He also serves as Emergency Preparedness Coordinator for the hospital and Chair of the Emergency Preparedness Committee.

As an early careerist, Aldrich worked as an administrative fellow for Trinity Health, and as a nuclear medicine chemist for the University of Michigan Health System.

Aldrich received his Bachelor of Science in biology and Master of Health Services Administration from the University of Michigan–Ann Arbor, as well as a Master of Business Administration from the University of Michigan–Dearborn. He is a member of the American College of Healthcare Executives (ACHE) and the Midwest Healthcare Executives Group and Associates (MHEGA).

Aldrich lives in Farmington Hills, Michigan, with his wife Melissa and daughter Abby.

fortunate to have had some of those profiled in this book as my own mentors and colleagues.

Climbing the Healthcare Management Ladder is organized into three sections: Success Factors, Managing Your Career, and Enhancing Your Success. Like the journey associated with one's life, the book generally flows along a path of what it takes to grow and be successful, how you go about personally achieving a successful career, and how you enhance and expand this success throughout the course of your career.

In the many forms of management and leadership work, we often hear that it is the journey that is most important, not so much the destination. The insights provided by the leaders in this book reveal a winding and often unpredictable course. It is the total collection of meaningful experiences that do much to shape a future leader; there are no clear predefined paths. Not everyone is cut out for the senior leadership CEO path. A future leader needs to constantly bring value to his or her organization as well as to the communities served. Across the spectrum of your career you must work hard, approach challenges with creativity and passion, and develop and build upon relationships.

For me, many echoes resonate from the interviews Jim conducted. Echoes of advice shared and advice received. Three findings of this work stand out the most. The first is to pursue your work with passion; the effort will be rewarded with opportunities that will refuel your passion. The second is the amazing similarity in insights these leaders provide into how to go about becoming successful. The important themes Jim identifies as contributors to success are shared across a diverse group of healthcare leaders. Lastly, the journey is unpredictable and will present you with unexpected changes, whether they are previously unanticipated opportunities or transitions of one's own making. Regarding the latter, I was struck by the number of leaders interviewed for this book who had made job and career changes based on self-reflection and adherence to their values. There are a number of examples of leaders who changed course, stepped back, and risked slowing their career progression due to conflicts with the leadership in their organizations regarding values and direction. "To thine own self be true" is also very much a part of the makeup of any leader. The self-awareness and self-confidence that allowed some of the leaders to momentarily step aside from their career progression undoubtedly contributed to the relatively rapid and subsequent continuance of their career successes.

The advice and insights shared by the leaders in this book will support you as you embark on your own journey into the field of health care. Their passion and commitment will inspire you to meet your own career leadership goals as well as speed your progress up the healthcare management ladder.

David A. Spivey
President and CEO, St. Mary Mercy Hospital

Introduction

When you look at the top of an organizational chart and see the Chief Executive Officer (CEO), have you ever wondered what it took for him or her to successfully climb the healthcare ladder? Was it luck, superior intelligence, being in the right place at the right time? Or rather was it a series of consistent habits, actions, and skills that assisted his or her climb? Imagine that you had 30 minutes of a CEO's undivided attention to ask how he or she made it to the top. You might ask questions such as Which specific actions or decisions led to your success? What experiences and skills are critical to obtain? Can you describe your mindset and how you feel it contributed to your success? In what ways were you vocal about your career goals? What would you do differently if you were just starting your career? What was the best career advice you ever received?

These questions and more swirled in my mind as I contemplated how I, too, could one day climb my way to the top. After endlessly searching the Internet and scanning numerous management books, it quickly became clear that there were no sources available that specifically addressed these types of questions for those of us working to climb the healthcare ladder. My search turned up many books that talked about rising to the CEO position in other industries, but not specifically in healthcare. I found books with titles such as *How to Think and Act Like a CEO, How To Be a CEO in Any Organization,*

How to Unleash Your Inner CEO, and even *How to Speak Like a CEO*. Despite this great variety of material, none of these books discussed the specific competencies and skills needed for successfully navigating the healthcare ladder.

With my search coming up empty, I decided instead to put into action some of the best career advice I have ever received: Find a job that you want to do, find who is doing that job, and find out what he or she did to get that job. Taking this advice to heart, I began to contact CEOs across the country in an effort to find answers to the questions that eluded me. In an effort to ensure that I left no stone unturned, I contacted and interviewed CEOs of health systems, academic medical centers, community hospitals, and critical access hospitals. I interviewed male and female CEOs as well as CEOs of for-profit and nonprofit hospitals. I spoke with CEOs who were at all stages of their careers, with some having been retired for several years and others who had just taken on their first CEO position. I interviewed CEOs who are members of the Modern Healthcare Hall of Fame, those who are listed among the 100 most powerful people in healthcare, and those who had received the American College of Healthcare Executive's Young Healthcare Executive of the Year award.

The CEOs who contributed to this book have the combined experience of more than 700 years of success working in all aspects of healthcare. They were all once in your shoes and have successfully climbed, and in some cases continue to climb, the healthcare ladder. Even if your ultimate goal is not to one day become a CEO, the advice, skills, and recommendations shared by these leaders will help encourage you to realize whatever level of success you desire. My hope is that this book will not only help you achieve your ultimate career goals, but also help prepare you to be successful once you attain them.

How This Book Can Help You

Each year the competition for jobs in healthcare administration grows more competitive. According to the American College of Healthcare Executives (ACHE), roughly 2,000 students each year receive a graduate degree in healthcare administration.[1] Programs are making it more convenient for a greater number of people to receive a graduate degree by offering options to take classes online and at night. Furthermore, due to economic uncertainty, workers are choosing to retire later in life, thus causing the pool of competent workers competing for a limited number of jobs to grow rapidly. Lastly, according to the U.S. Department of Labor, jobs in the healthcare field have been estimated to grow by 22.5% between 2008 and 2018, which will continue to attract a growing number of workers from other industries. The competition for jobs in the field of healthcare is intensifying and, therefore, successful career planning is more critical than ever before.

Preparing for the intense competition that lies ahead of you and learning from the advice of mentors who have gone before you will be vital to your success. Have you ever had a great mentor who had a wealth of experience, always gave you outstanding advice, and seemed to have just the right answer to all of your questions? Does a mentor such as this even exist? If you are one of the lucky few to answer yes, then hold on to that person and continue to learn from his or her knowledge and experience. Most of you, however, will have likely answered no, because these sages are certainly in short supply. The bottom line is that it is impossible to expect any one person to have all the answers and to have done and tried everything in his or her career.

My goal is that as you read this book, you will have 29 mentors who are all CEOs and who are all telling you exactly what made them successful and how you can find similar success. It is important to note that this book provides no shortcuts, quick fixes, or magic bullets to achieve success in your career, simply for the fact that there are none. The advice from the CEOs in this book addresses the skills, actions, and techniques that when consistently applied will help mold you into a successful healthcare executive. No one person has all the answers and no two careers are exactly the same. What may have worked for one person may not work in your situation. For this reason it is important that you receive advice from as many different sources as possible and begin to adopt and apply the advice that resonates the most with you. This book draws on advice from numerous CEOs who have a variety of different backgrounds and experiences. You will come to notice that there is not a consensus on one ideal career path or even what is the best job to take right out of graduate school. It all really comes down to who you are, what experiences you have had, and how hard you are willing to work. As you read this book you will learn that there are general actions, habits, and skills that when consistently applied will lead you to success time and time again, regardless of the situation, environment, or circumstance.

One of my favorite quotes in this regard is "We become what we want to be by consistently being what we want to become."[2]

By consistently applying the advice from the CEOs in this book and by consistently being who you want to become, you will begin to develop yourself into a successful executive. This process will not happen overnight, but anything worth having never comes easy. Furthermore, you should not wait until you are a director to begin influencing and leading others or until you are a vice president to begin developing strategies or until you are a CEO to begin thinking about the "big picture." You need to begin modeling and applying the skills today of the job you want tomorrow. It really is a classic which-came-first scenario, the chicken or the egg? The same is true with your career. Why would someone hire you to be a CEO if you have no experience being a CEO? But how can you get experience being a CEO if no one is willing to hire you? The solution is you need to gain experience doing CEO-like duties before you get the job to prove that you can do the job. This model does not only apply to a CEO position, but also to any position throughout your career. Becoming a successful and competent leader happens by consistently being who you want to become, day after day.

The Road to Competence

As you learn and apply the advice in this book, my hope is that it will become a part of who you become as a leader. My goal is to move you from being an Unconscious Incompetent leader to an Unconscious Competent leader (see figure). The Conscious Competence Ladder shows that at first as you embark on your career path you are an Unconscious Incompetent leader, meaning that you simply do not yet know what you do not know to succeed. As you begin to identify the experiences, knowledge, and skills you will need to develop and succeed in your career, you then move up to becoming a Conscious Incompetent leader. You next become a Conscious Competent leader who is aware of your new skillsets and is working toward refining them. Finally, as your skillsets and experiences become habitual and you perform them with greater ease, less conscious effort, and more confidence, you become an Unconscious Competent leader.[3] As you consistently practice and begin to internalize the techniques and strategies in this book, you will eventually begin to demonstrate them unconsciously and they will become a part of who you are as a leader.

As you look at the CEO position at the top of the organizational chart and ask yourself how one day you, too, can get there, my hope is

The Conscious Competence Ladder

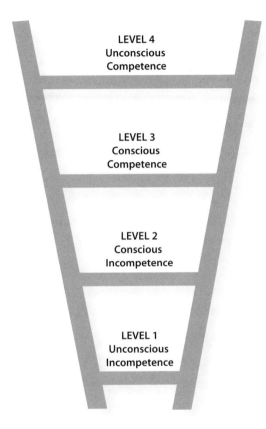

LEVEL 4
Unconscious
Competence

LEVEL 3
Conscious
Competence

LEVEL 2
Conscious
Incompetence

LEVEL 1
Unconscious
Incompetence

that once you have finished this book you will not be asking how you can get there, but rather how anyone can stop you from getting there. A journey of a thousand miles begins with a single step, and let me be the first to say "congratulations" on taking that first step!

Success Factors

My reason for writing this book was to discover what "success factors" assisted the CEOs in their climb up the healthcare management ladder, as well as to offer advice on how others can apply these factors in their own careers.

I began my journey by asking the CEOs a variety of general and open-ended questions, including

What characteristics and actions helped you achieve your success?

What did you not learn in graduate school that you wish you knew?

What is the best advice you have ever received?

If you could go back, what would you do differently?

I purposely asked vague and open-ended questions because I wanted each CEO to reflect on the specific factors that contributed to his or her career success. Asking these types of questions also encouraged the CEOs to provide a variety of responses covering numerous topics, thoughts, and ideas, without any influence or prompting from me to identify specific skills or traits. I fought the urge to provide additional guidance as they reflected on and shared their many experiences and accomplishments. My efforts to avoid imparting my own bias into the interviews proved fruitful in that I received very specific and personal advice on what success factors each CEO felt were critical to his or her success.

I had assumed that the CEOs' responses might vary based on their age, types of organizations they worked in, and even their gender. I was surprised to find that, in fact, the complete opposite turned out to be true. As I interviewed more and more of the CEOs, I quickly began to see amazing similarities in all of their responses, regardless of their background, age, gender, experience, or any other characteristic that differentiated them.

The key success factors that the CEOs discussed are strikingly similar and began to fall into the following five themes:

1. Jump at and create your opportunities
2. Work hard and work smart
3. Relationships are key
4. Variety equals success
5. Learn the business

These themes were consistently present in all of the CEOs' answers and served as the broad, overarching contributing factors to their success. As you read this book and learn more about these success factors, continually ask yourself how you can begin to apply them consistently in your own career.

1

Getting Started

If you could look 20 years into the future and see where you are in your career, I think many of you would be surprised by what you saw. You probably would never have guessed where you ended up and all the twists and turns that your career took. Your career path may not have gone the way you planned, and maybe your ideal path turned out not to be so ideal. It's a given that there will be unforeseen events and variability in life; nevertheless, it's important to have at least some idea of what direction you want your career to go.

You may be a student or early careerist and have known from day one that you wanted to pursue a career in healthcare administration. Alternatively, you may be well into your career only to have discovered that you've gone down a path that wasn't right for you. Regardless of which group you fall into, thinking about and planning for your career is always time well spent. It's estimated that a person will change careers five to seven times in his or her lifetime.[4] While there is much debate about what actually constitutes a "career change" and how these numbers are tracked, the point is that you will likely change jobs and careers more than once. Whatever situation you're in, you can rest assured that you're not alone and that others have been in your shoes. The CEOs interviewed for this book have navigated through similar waters and have found successful and fulfilling careers.

The good news is that the fact you are reading this book shows you have at least drawn some conclusions about what you want to do and in what direction you want to move your career. Of course, your plans can always change, which reminds me of a quote from singer Jon Bon Jovi: "Map out your future, but do it in pencil." I'm also reminded of another quote from screenwriter and director Kevin Smith: "Sometimes the path you're on is not as important as the direction you're heading." The key point to understand is that your career isn't going to follow a straight line and your specific job titles and responsibilities will vary from other people's experiences. Ultimately, however, with hard work and determination, you'll arrive at your destination.

As part of the interviews, the first question I asked each CEO was "Did you start out your career wanting to be a CEO and, if not, at what point in your career did you decide that this was what you wanted to do?" My reasoning for asking this question first was to try and understand each CEO's mindset and determine at what point he or she began to actively strive for the position of CEO. My interviews showed that 11 of the 29 CEOs began their career with this goal in mind, while the other 18 said that they had not explicitly thought about becoming a CEO. Rather, their motivation and goal was simply to become a leader in healthcare and to have a positive impact.

Two responses really capture the feelings of all the CEOs I interviewed:

> I knew that I wanted to be in healthcare, but starting out I didn't know that I wanted to be a CEO. I wanted to be in leadership and management, and once I knew that, everything else fell into place. (Sean Williams, President and CEO, Mercy Medical Center)

> I didn't set out to be a CEO, but rather I wanted to occupy a senior position in the field where I could have a significant impact on my organization and the community at the same time. (Tom Priselac, President and CEO, Cedars-Sinai Health System)

Regardless of whether they started out their careers knowing that they wanted to be a CEO or simply to make a difference, they all expressed that a career in healthcare was in line with their core values and that serving others was the major driver behind their decision to enter into the field.

As I mentioned earlier, people will change their jobs and careers many times in their lifetime, and the CEOs in this book are no exception. For example, Jack Weiner (President and CEO, St. Joseph Mercy Hospital–Oakland) began his career as a clinical pharmacist. Frustrated with what he was seeing and with his inability to affect what was impacting him as a pharmacist, Jack ultimately decided that "I needed to go and sit in the chair where change happens." Quint Studer (President and CEO, Studer Group) spent the first 10 years of his career working as a special education teacher before taking a job as a community relations representative in a substance abuse hospital. When Mike Slubowski (President and CEO, Sisters of Charity of Leavenworth Health System) started his career, he hadn't even thought he was going to work in healthcare. He initially worked in the auto industry as an accountant, but eventually his job was downsized. It was only by chance that Mike ended up in the finance division of Henry Ford Health System. Kathleen Griffiths (retired, President and CEO, Chelsea Community Hospital) began her career as a first grade teacher and then became a social worker in a psychiatric hospital for children. The hospital kept asking her to do more and more administrative work, and soon Kathleen found that she liked the duties more so than the clinical work. Phil McCorkle (President and CEO,

> " I needed to go and sit in the chair where change happens. "

St. Mary's Health Care) wanted to be a researcher (at Wake Forest he majored in biology and minored in chemistry). As he spent more and more time in these areas of study, he decided that he didn't like the research aspect and that it wasn't going to be the right career path for him. During his studies Phil happened to take a course on hospital administration and said it was phenomenal. He decided to change fields and chose instead to pursue a master's degree in hospital administration. Alan Channing (President and CEO, Sinai Health System) spent time working for an engineering consultant, the federal government, and Mack Trucks before finally focusing on health services administration. Alan shared with me that working in a hospital setting really feels like home and that it's a place where he can apply his interests and make a difference in people's lives.

Other CEOs I interviewed started in healthcare but had no plans to pursue an administrative career path. Rick O'Connell (Executive Vice President and COO, Hospital Networks for Trinity Health) began his career in healthcare at the age of 16 working as an orderly to give him something to do during the summers. Betty Noyes (President, Noyes & Associates, Ltd.) always wanted to make a difference in healthcare and began her career as a nurse. Bob Milewski (Senior Vice President, Hospital Relations, Blue Cross Blue Shield of Michigan) started by working in a pharmacy, became a student pharmacist, and then ultimately developed an interest in the management side of the business. Rob Casalou (President and CEO, St. Joseph Mercy Hospitals–Ann Arbor, Livingston) initially wanted to be a doctor, but quickly realized that it wasn't going to happen for him once he began his premed classes. He decided instead that if he was going to get into healthcare, he would have to get there a different way.

From these varied backgrounds and experiences, it's clear that there isn't one single path to follow and that you can start your career in a multitude of different areas and still find success. As Quint Studer shared with me:

> I feel that 98 percent of people in healthcare took certain jobs and then eventually they were put into a supervisory role. Most people don't start out wanting to be an executive, they do good work and then are promoted and continue to take on more and more responsibility.

The fact that you are reading this book shows that you are committed to maximizing your career as a healthcare leader and want to make a significant impact on your organization and community. That said, it's important to understand that circumstances have changed a lot since the CEOs in this book were first coming up the healthcare ladder. Mike Slubowski notes that there are challenges with how leadership development and mentoring is done today that are inhibiting some of the opportunities for people climbing the ladder:

> Back when I started my career it was very customary for people in fellowships to end up being recruited into an assistant administrator job right out of their fellowship. Also people would take big chances with you if they felt you had the raw material and would give you big responsibilities.

Mike adds that another challenge people face today is that healthcare has gotten much more complex, competitive, and financially focused. "We tend to find much narrower functional roles for people to take on, and unless there is someone continually mentoring them and working on career development with them, there is a tendency for people to get pigeonholed," he explains. Another difference from when Mike was coming up the ladder is that employers today are not, for whatever reason, willing to take as much of a risk on someone by giving the person challenging assignments. When he was at Henry Ford they took a big chance on him when he was asked to run a clinic and then again when he was asked to open other clinics. Within a short period of time Mike took on the responsibility of managing all of the sites as well as building new ones. "Basically, I was learning on the go," he says.

Don Wegmiller (Chairman and CEO, C-Suite Resources), who began his career back in the early 1960s, best illustrates how much the field of healthcare has changed. According to Don, back then the only positions available were either that of hospital CEO or one of the assistant positions. Don notes, "Pretty much everybody who entered graduate school at that time expected that they would become a CEO." He says that this was largely because in the early 1960s having a graduate degree in healthcare administration was relatively rare and so this was the degree that hospital boards and other hospital managers were looking for. "It

> Some opportunities are in hospitals, some are in systems, and some are in physician groups. There's such a span of options now.

was a lot simpler and easier, and the expectation of becoming a CEO was a lot higher," Don says. This expectation wasn't unique to Don, who recalls that in his graduating class of about 20 students roughly 75 percent of them believed they one day would become a hospital CEO.

Recognizing that opportunities have changed greatly, Don Wegmiller also notes that for people today, interesting, challenging, and rewarding opportunities in healthcare are multitudes greater than when he was coming up:

> It is no longer the 'end all, be all' to be a hospital CEO since there are so many career opportunities available now in healthcare, and I think this change has been for the better. Some opportunities are in hospitals, some are in systems, and some are in physician groups. There's such a span of options now that fit a lot of different people's aspirations and interests.

Similarly, David Fine (President and CEO, St. Luke's Episcopal Health System) says that what was true 35 years ago when he started up the ladder and what's true today are very different:

In 1974 when I started, if you had performed reasonably well in graduate school and reasonably well in your post-graduate residency, then there was a much better than even chance that you were going to start out your career as either an assistant administrator or at a vice president level, depending on the titling system used by the organization. Today it can easily take 10 years to work your way up from a job of much narrower scope to such a position.

David says that opportunities have changed quite a bit as the field has matured and as the number of graduates has grown.

———————————

From the CEOs' comments it's clear that your career path will not follow a straight line and that you can start in any number of areas or industries and still find success in the field of healthcare. It's also important to understand that the field has changed a lot from when many of the CEOs of today were coming up the ladder, and that it will take longer periods of time for those now beginning their careers to obtain senior management positions. This should not be viewed as a negative or hindrance, because the field of healthcare is more complex and demanding than ever before. Additionally, a vast array of opportunities exists in healthcare today and the potential to develop a much richer and broader scope of experiences is magnitudes greater than ever before. So as you think about where you will be in your career in the next 5, 10, or 20 years, don't focus on the specific job, but rather on what overarching skills and experiences you want to have in your toolkit. Continue to follow your career path no matter how many twists, turns, and detours you run into along the way, and remember this quote from Zig Ziglar: "Where you start is not as important as where you finish."

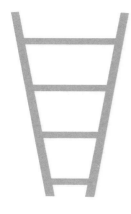

CLIMBING TOOLS
Getting Started

- Your career won't follow a straight line and your specific job titles and responsibilities will vary from other people's experiences. With hard work and determination, however, you'll arrive at your destination.

- Healthcare and serving others are in line with the core values of the CEOs and were the major drivers in their decision to enter into the field.

- There isn't one path to follow; you can start your career in a multitude of different areas and still find success in the healthcare field.

- Continually work on developing the skills and experiences you'll need in your career to avoid being pigeonholed into a narrow functional role.

Climbing the Healthcare Management Ladder: Career Advice from the Top on How to Succeed, by Jim Aldrich (Copyright © 2013, by Health Professors Press, Inc.)

2

Jump at and Create Your Opportunities

One success factor that is common among the CEOs is that they didn't just sit back and wait for people to hand them opportunities. Rather, they consistently looked for ways to learn new skills and gain experience in different areas. The shared message is that no one is going to manage your career for you and so you need to be proactive in looking for opportunities to develop skills and experience that will contribute to your success. No one is going to say to you, "Well it looks like you haven't had experience doing 'X,' so let's move you into that department," or "You've been doing your current job for a while, so let's move you to another department so you can get some additional experiences." In an ideal world, these types of conversations would be taking place with your supervisor, but in the real world growing your skillset and gaining new knowledge and experience is going to be all up to you. This could require, for example, applying for an open position in a new area, volunteering to be on a hospital committee, or even offering to take on additional duties and tasks that are above and beyond your current job requirements and that no one else is willing to do. To be a successful leader you'll need to have a broad exposure to many different areas, and you'll need to actively look for ways to develop a range of experience in any way you can.

A key principle that really speaks to playing an active role in building your own success is the 20/80 Principle of Performance from the book, *The 5 Patterns of Extraordinary Careers*, by James Citrin and Richard Smith. According to the authors, 80% of a job offers little chance for differentiation, is narrowly defined by a specific job description, and on the surface is quite inflexible. The authors explain that

> It is the ability to get beyond merely achieving what others want you to do and break through to deliver unanticipated impact that will give you and your company the most return, creating results that can truly distinguish you. Unlike the 80/20 principle in business, it is usually the last 20 percent of what you accomplish beyond your predefined objectives that allows you to truly differentiate yourself. . . . The reality is that you can do what you are told at work and do a good job of it and still not have success or security in your position.[5]

Whatever tasks you do within the 80% that constitutes your specific job description will be viewed as "just doing your job," and successful completion of these tasks will not separate you from others as being a "star" or "exceptional" employee. The key point is that every job has some discretionary time and this time makes up the remaining 20% of your job. This is the block of time you can use to really excel in your career or remain stagnant. During this 20% block of time most people just continue to perform the standard tasks that make up the required 80% of their job. The really successful people, however, use this discretionary time to their advantage by seeking out additional exposure and access to new experiences. They use this time to think about what they could do to make their boss's job easier and then do it without waiting for permission. They efficiently accomplish the required 80% of their job and then take on additional tasks and assignments nobody else wants to do or has the time to do. These people reach out beyond their predefined job description and jump at and create their own opportunities to achieve success for themselves.

> [E]specially when you're starting your career, you just don't say no, and you jump at every opportunity you can.

Throughout Jack Weiner's career he would always look for ways to gain unique experiences that would set him apart from others: "I was always willing to step out of the box and do the things that other people didn't want to do. I sought out opportunities and when something came up I was the first person to say that's interesting, let me give that a shot." When other people would ask "What is that?" Jack would say,

"Let me do it!" Similar to Jack's experience, Carrie Owen Plietz (CEO, Sutter Medical Center–Sacramento) would also try to take advantage of the opportunities that came her way:

> You never say no. Of course, you have to be reasonable about this, but especially when you're starting your career, you just don't say no, and you jump at every opportunity you can. If the door opens, make sure you're there and you are willing to go for it, because it's amazing how those cracks in the door and those opportunities can then lead to something even greater.

Nancy Schlichting (CEO, Henry Ford Health System) took the same initiative as part of her career progression:

> I looked at my career in terms of what I was doing at each moment and then tried to take full advantage of the opportunities for learning and growth. I always had the feeling that if I did my job really well and people saw the value I was adding to the organization, then I would have opportunities come my way. Then when opportunities came in front of me, I typically jumped at them. If you really want to advance, you've got to take some risks and you've got to try and do things maybe before you're completely ready. So when things came my way, I did them.

In terms of doing things that maybe you're not completely ready for, David Olson (Chief Strategy Officer and Senior Vice President, Froedtert Health System) shared with me a story of when he jumped at an opportunity before he had full knowledge of the subject matter. David had been working at St. Joseph's of Marshfield in Wisconsin for about 2 months when the system CEO stopped by the hospital and told the leadership team that they had just received a request for proposal (RFP) from a critical access hospital to have a health system acquire them. The critical access hospital had sent the RFP to two other health systems and so this was going to be a competitive situation. The CEO of the health system that David was working in asked if anybody knew how to prepare and respond to an RFP and how to get the critical access hospital to ultimately accept their proposal. David said, "I really didn't know how to do this, although I had been indirectly involved in similar work at St. Luke's in Cedar Rapids." He raised his hand and accepted the challenge: "No one else in the room knew how to do this, so my limited knowledge actually made me something of an expert. As a result, we ended up being successful in the acquisition and I ended up serving as the CEO for one year." By being willing to jump at an opportunity, despite not having extensive knowledge in an area and essentially "learning on the go," David was able to demonstrate his abilities to successfully lead a challenging project and subsequently secured his first CEO position. Although the task was challenging and he didn't have a lot of experience in the area of RFPs, neither did anyone else in the group. David was basically in a no-lose situation and, regardless of what the final outcome was, the fact that no one else had experience allowed the expectation of success to be set low. Had David failed, it would have been chalked up to the fact that no one had experience in acquiring another hospital and so the group failed due to inexperience. But because David ended up being successful, the opportunity became a résumé-enhancing experience as well as a turning point in his career.

> If you really want to advance, you've got to take some risks and you've got to try and do things maybe before you're completely ready.

In addition to jumping at opportunities, it's also important to be ready for the unexpected opportunities that might be thrust upon you. One day while working as the Director of Oncology at Providence Hospital in Southfield, Michigan, Rob Casalou was sitting at his desk when his boss walked up and asked: "Rob, we just bought a lab. It's going to be a tough merger and I know you're running Oncology, but I thought of you and we'd like to have you merge this lab into the organization. Do you want to take it on?" Rob knew that this would be a good opportunity to gain new experience and so he decided to take on the challenge. "I always tried to be visible," he says, "but not in an overt way like a little dog yipping at the big dog's heels, but rather by just being present, being enthusiastic, and being willing to take anything on and then getting results." Rob always made sure that he delivered on everything he did and then let the results speak for themselves. It was because of the great job he was doing running the Oncology Department that Rob was asked to take on the lab merger. And after successfully merging the lab into the organization, he was subsequently given new responsibilities. So with each successful project, Rob was able to add to his credibility and move his career forward.

It might seem easy to simply jump at every opportunity that comes your way and dive head first into areas where you have no experience and believe that it will all work out in the end. For most people, however, this can be a scary and uncomfortable path. The truth is that taking on new challenges in unfamiliar areas takes courage and requires you to be unafraid of failure. As Phil McCorkle says, "You need to do things that are outside of your comfort zone, and you really are only as good as you push or stretch yourself." This brings us back to the chicken–egg scenario that I mentioned earlier: How can you get the job if you don't yet have the experience, but how can you get the experience if you've never done the job? The answer is that you either need to find ways to perform the duties of the job you want before you officially have the job, or you can take a risk and try and convince others that you can do the job despite having no previous experience.

Nancy Schlichting did just that while working at Akron City Hospital in Ohio. She took a big risk and it paid off for her. Throughout her career Nancy took advantage of many opportunities in which she had little clue how to do the job, but she decided to stick her neck out anyway because she knew they were great chances to enhance her experience and further her career. She became the Chief Operating Officer (COO) at Akron City Hospital, a 650-bed teaching hospital in Ohio, with only 1 year of experience in Operations and 2 years of experience in Strategic Planning. Nancy said,

> I wrote a letter to Al Gilbert, who was the CEO at the time, and told him all of my ideas about how I could be the COO and how we would work together and create a great vision for the organization. Al will tell you even to this day that if I hadn't written that letter, he would never have considered me for the job because I was so young and inexperienced.

At the time Nancy was only 28 years old, while all of her peers were in their 50s. Nancy created a great opportunity for herself by writing a letter to the CEO and having the courage to accept the position of COO with only 1 year of operations experience.

David Stark (President and CEO/Executive Vice President, Blank Children's Hospital/Iowa Health–Des Moines) had a similar experience to Nancy's and is probably the most striking example of seizing a huge opportunity without having a lot of previous experience when he was promoted from Administrative Fellow to interim CEO at the age of only 25. David completed his master's in healthcare administration at the University of Iowa and then took a fellowship position with Iowa Health in Des Moines. During his fellowship, the CEO of the rural Clarke County Hospital in Osceola suddenly quit, and David said that there were no obvious replacements. David's boss asked if he would step in and run the hospital. David recalls, "It was the opportunity of a lifetime to jump in and run something. So I commuted 47 miles down the interstate every day for 7 months. I knew I must have done a halfway decent job, because they wanted me to stay." I asked David what he did early in his fellowship to demonstrate to people that he was capable of assuming the role of interim CEO at such a young age:

> When I first started my fellowship I never turned anything down. I said yes to every project and opportunity no matter if it was really small and seemingly trivial. People said, 'Hey, he's willing to work hard and step right in,' and I think that made an impression.

It may seem a little unrealistic in today's environment for a 28-year-old with 1 year of operations experience to become the COO of a 650-bed hospital or for a 25-year-old to go straight from administrative fellow to interim CEO, but the fact is Nancy and David were proactive in making it happen for themselves and you, too, can do the same. The advice and example they give are important because sometimes we hold ourselves back due to self-doubt, preconceived notions, fear of the unknown, fear of failing, fear of looking foolish, and the list goes on and on. The key point is that you need to be willing to take risks and embrace new challenges. This is true no matter what age you are or how long you've been in your career. One of my favorite sayings is "Nothing ventured, nothing gained." If you always stay in your comfort zone, then that's where you're always going to be. I liken this to lifting weights: If you lift the same weight day after day, your muscles eventually grow to a certain point, and then they stop growing. In other words, they don't have any reason or need to grow any larger than they already are. It's only once you begin to increase the weight that your muscles are forced out of stagnation and begin to grow. The same holds true for your career; unless you are consistently seeking out new "weights" or "opportunities," you will never grow as a leader and achieve your full potential.

The best way to create more opportunities for yourself is to take on projects, tasks, and roles that nobody else has shown an interest in taking on. This will be easy to do, because there will be no competition for these jobs, and your request to get involved and help will surely be welcomed with open arms. This is exactly what all of the CEOs did throughout their careers, which allowed them to become known as the "go-to" person in their respective organizations. Carrie Owen Plietz says that by taking on challenges that maybe nobody else wants, and then hitting them "out of the park," people will notice and will potentially come to you again the next time something else comes up. Additionally, when I asked Garry Faja (President and CEO, St. Joseph Mercy Health System–Southeastern Michigan region) if there were any areas that should be avoided, he simply responded, "No, you should take on anything." He notes that sometimes those climbing the ladder will be given the jobs that nobody else wants and their boss might say, "Why don't you be in charge of volunteers?" or "Why don't you coordinate with the medical staff auxiliary?" or "Maybe you could take on the library?" Garry adds that, "Despite what you are given, always do the best you can."

The CEOs who were interviewed for this book certainly did the best they could throughout their careers, and they consistently looked for ways to learn new skills and gain exposure to different areas. They did not simply sit back and wait for others to guide their careers; they took their careers into their own hands and created opportunities for themselves. Doing so allowed them to gain a wide range of experience and to become the go-to person in their organization. As you also look for ways to jump at and create opportunities in your own career, you will begin to build a foundation of skills and experience that will allow you to be a successful leader for many years to come.

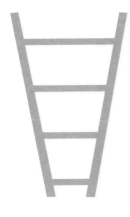

CLIMBING TOOLS

Jump at and Create Your Opportunities

- Don't just sit back and wait for people to hand you opportunities. Rather, consistently look for ways to learn new skills and gain experience in different areas.

- Follow the 20/80 Principle of Performance: use the 20% of discretionary time at work to take on additional tasks and assignments to create results that can truly distinguish you.

- Reach out beyond your predefined job description and jump at and create your own opportunities.

- If you want to advance, you've got to take some risks by taking on opportunities that you might not be completely ready for. The opportunity may become a résumé-enhancing experience as well as a turning point in your career.

- Always be ready to take on unexpected opportunities that might be thrust upon you.

- Taking on new challenges in unfamiliar areas will take courage and require you not to be afraid of failure.

- Become known as the "go-to" person in your organization by taking on projects, tasks, and roles that nobody else wants, which will allow you to acquire new skills and experiences.

Climbing the Healthcare Management Ladder: Career Advice from the Top on How to Succeed, by Jim Aldrich (Copyright © 2013, by Health Professors Press, Inc.)

3

Work Hard and
Work Smart

Another success factor the CEOs share is that hard work and sacrifice were keys to their success. This comes as no surprise. You've probably heard countless times that "You reap what you sow," or "A job worth doing is a job worth doing right," or "There is no substitute for hard work." While these expressions might seem overly simplistic and even clichéd, they're nevertheless true and valid. Regardless of each CEO's level of intelligence, charisma, or experience, hard work was at the foundation of everything he or she achieved. Thomas Jefferson once said, "I'm a great believer in luck, and I find that the harder I work, the more I have of it." I love this quote, and I'm a big believer that we can play a significant role in shaping our own destiny by deciding to work hard. Simply stated, hard work can lead to better outcomes and consistent success as well as open doors to unforeseen opportunities, which to others may appear to be due solely to "luck."

While hard work is obviously good and beneficial for your career, the CEOs stressed that the combination of *working hard* and *working smart* is what will really maximize your time, talent, and energy. It's important to understand that working hard and working smart are two very different concepts. The following is one of the best explanations I've found that speaks to the distinction:

> People who work hard and people who work smart have different measures of success. Those that work hard usually evaluate success based on

inputs such as the number of hours they work and the number of tasks they accomplish in a day or in a week. . . . Typically, hard work means something like 60 or 70 hours a week . . . , working at home in the evenings and weekends, and continuously juggling multiple projects in a frantic attempt to get them all done. This is not hard work, this is simply poor management of your time and . . . the inability to balance your work life and your personal life.

Those who work smart usually evaluate success based on the amount of discretionary time they have to do whatever it is they want to do. Smart workers don't focus on inputs, they focus on prioritizing in order to achieve the most valuable outputs in the most efficient ways. Smart workers usually have much better work–life balance, are able to identify their strengths and weaknesses, and manage time effectively. For example, a smart worker will realize that they are more productive during a certain time of day and will batch their tasks based on difficulty to match with when they are the most productive.[6]

In other words, the difference between working hard and working smart comes down to how you define and measure success. So the question you should be asking yourself is, "How do I define and measure success?" Is it from producing complicated spreadsheets, generating lots of data, and working more hours than everyone else? Or rather is it from determining the key outputs and only producing the information that will provide the greatest results? However you define and measure success, it's critical to remember that working hard has its benefits, but when combined with working smart, your level of success will increase tenfold.

Too much of a good thing can be counterproductive and can even lead to a false sense of security. Such is the case with only working smart and failing also to work hard. According to Jon Gordon, author of *Training Camp: What the Best Do Better Than Everyone Else*:

> It's true that by working smarter and being more productive with your time you may not have to work as hard to enjoy your current level of success. But if you want to be more successful or rise to the top of your field, then "smarter, not harder" won't do. Those who adopt the motto of working smarter, not harder, will eventually be left in the dust by the competition. The best are always striving to get better. They are always pushing themselves beyond their comfort zone. They are always innovating and improving.[7]

The key point to understand is that simply working hard without a defined purpose or goal will result in a lot of work being done that may or may not actually achieve your desired objective. Also, simply working smart might allow you to get things done faster and more efficiently, but if you then spend the extra time you have gained on other unproductive tasks, then the ultimate benefit is lost. Thus it is important that you work both hard and smart at everything you do throughout your career. The 29 CEOs understood this concept early in their careers, and it played a major role in the achievement of their success.

Early on Kevin Unger (President and CEO, Poudre Valley Hospital) knew he wanted to pursue a career in hospital administration and that to get his foot in the door he needed to develop real-life experience working in hospital operations. He was willing to work both hard and smart to find ways to gain the experience. Never having worked in a hospital before, Kevin decided that he would sacrifice some of his free time by volunteering at the University of Colorado Hospital while he was in graduate school. He subsequently secured a position as a volunteer with the hospital's vice president of operations. This opportunity certainly wasn't the typical volunteer position of passing out magazines, filling blanket warmers, and greeting visitors. And you may even be thinking to yourself that Kevin "lucked out," and that the vice president of operations at your local hospital would never take a student volunteer (they're too busy, don't have the time, and already have enough people vying for their attention). My response is, well, have you asked? Do you know this for sure? The earlier quote from Thomas Jefferson rings true here, in that the harder you work the more luck you'll have. Although I recognize that there was probably a bit of luck involved with Kevin getting this volunteer position, the key point is that he was willing to sacrifice his free time and thus put himself in a position to create his own luck.

> "I've always been willing to step up to the plate, to take on a new challenge or a new responsibility and never give up. It's all about having a basis toward action."

As a volunteer, Kevin wasn't getting paid and he certainly had many other things he could have been doing with his free time. He took the opportunity, however, to work hard and as a result put himself in a position to learn about the day-to-day operational components of the hospital. Kevin notes that, "In this day and age with the job market the way it is, you have to be willing to volunteer and get in there and get some experience that you can put on your résumé that will differentiate you from other candidates." Kevin knew that his volunteer experience would eventually pay off down the road and that working smart would give him the competitive advantage he needed to get his foot in the door and differentiate himself from others.

Make Your Experiences Count

Similar to Kevin Unger, Nancy Schlichting knew that getting experience any way she could would be of great benefit and help open doors throughout her career. Some of the most important jobs that Nancy has held were the ones she had before she went to graduate school. Nancy earned a bachelor's in public policy from Duke University but decided after graduating that she really wanted to pursue a career in hospital administration. Despite having a degree from Duke, Nancy chose to take jobs that were very low-paying and often had no health benefits simply to get experience and to learn more about hospital operations. She worked in cancer outreach at Duke University Hospital in the radiation oncology department and as an assistant on several nursing units. She even worked as a switchboard operator on the weekends. Nancy says, "I got paid $3.25 an hour with no benefits and I did this despite having a degree from Duke. I did all of this to get frontline experience and to gain an understanding of hospital operations from the ground level."

Nancy certainly worked hard and was smart about the types of jobs she took. She didn't simply work to earn a paycheck; rather, she knew what her end goal was and took jobs that would function as stepping stones to achieving her career objectives. Additionally, she was willing to make the sacrifice of earning less money to gain the key experiences that would carry her throughout her career. Nancy's "smart work" paid off because during graduate school she was hired as an intern at Sloan Kettering Memorial Cancer Center in New York City:

> This internship experience was only possible because of the prior experiences I had from working in the Radiation Oncology department at Duke University Hospital. Having worked with cancer patients and

having had these types of experiences showed the internship selection committee that I had a high level of maturity and a strong work ethic. So these were very important decisions that I made early in my career.

Kevin Unger shared the story of how their incoming administrative fellow at Poudre Valley Hospital for 2010 applied the concept of working hard and smart. What impressed Kevin and his colleagues the most about this candidate was that during the previous summer he had planned to do an internship at the Mayo Clinic in Phoenix, Arizona. The position was all set and the Mayo Clinic was going to pay him as well as take care of his housing. The clinic's budget, however, was tightened and the internship position was eliminated for 2009. The candidate decided to go ahead with the internship despite not being paid, to gain the experience he felt he needed. This really impressed the interviewing committee at Poudre Valley Hospital and it played a large part in their decision to ultimately choose him later for a fellowship. Kevin says, "Doing things like this, and being willing to take on any project, and being that go-to person who is willing to take on projects that may not be glamorous and then hitting them out of the ballpark are the types of things that will set you apart." The candidate certainly set himself apart from others by being willing to take on the unglamorous role of an unpaid intern while all of his peers were earning a salary. His decision to work both hard and smart opened doors to unforeseen opportunities and directly contributed to being awarded a paid fellowship the year following his internship.

> " When you look at people who are successful, they work hard and put in the time to be successful. "

Working Hard Requires Passion

Working hard and working smart also mean that you have passion for the work you're doing and that you deliver on the projects and assignments that are assigned to you. Rick O'Connell's father always taught him that no matter what the job is, you do the best you can and never stop until you get it done. His father also taught him that failures will occur and it's how you recover from your failures that will determine your success. Rick's father was right—your level of success really comes down to your attitude and your passion for the work you're performing. Rick's personal formula for success is "A-cubed B.T.A.," which stands for *Attitude, Attitude, Attitude* and a *Basis Toward Action*. He adds that

> The status quo is so prevalent in hospitals, and we're creatures of doing the same thing over and over again, because it's the way we've always done it. So you've got to have a basis toward change or a basis toward taking action. A lot of times we are really hesitant to do something, but my attitude has always been to just do it, and if it doesn't work then we'll change it as we go. At least we're changing and always moving in a positive direction. It's all about attitude, because how you face your work each and every day, how you look at the diversity that comes your way, and how you celebrate the successes is all about your attitude toward your work, and your attitude is the most important thing.

Rick feels that some people have the drive and some people don't, and that it comes down to what's inside someone as to whether they have the fortitude and willingness to keep pressing on. Rick said that it's similar to how scientists come up with great discoveries; if they just quit, humankind would never advance. Rather, they press on trying to understand more and more so that we as a whole can excel. Rick explains,

> The same thing is true for a career in healthcare. You've just got to have that fortitude to just keep pushing, keep asking questions, and be willing to do the things that you normally don't want to do. I've always been willing to step up to the plate, to take on a new challenge or a new responsibility and never give up. It's all about having a basis toward action.

Having passion for your work also involves going to great lengths to pay attention to the details of what you're doing. Peter Karadjoff (President, Providence Park Hospital) recommends that

> When you're working on a project for someone, don't wow them just to try to wow them, but rather wow them with the details, wow them with great follow through, and wow them by giving them more than they asked for when they first met with you.

Similarly, Nancy Schlichting recalls that "I always went to a very deep level whenever I was given an assignment. A lot of my peers would take the easy approach, but I always tried to do my homework thoroughly and I worked harder than anyone else." Nancy says that her work ethic, the hours she kept, her level of commitment, and the way she related to the people she worked with were the keys to her success.

Speaking to the importance of having a strong work ethic, Dave Spivey (President and CEO, St. Mary Mercy Hospital) says that for many executives there can be a tendency to sometimes make your private and family life secondary to your professional career, and it's important to maintain balance in both areas. He adds that

> Having said that, though, I think it's hard work that often gets you ahead. When you look at people who are successful, they work hard and put in the time to be successful. One of the people I was fortunate to have been exposed to was Gail Warden [President Emeritus, Henry Ford Health System], who was a tremendously hard worker. I remember meeting with him at 6:00 in the morning at Henry Ford Hospital, and he would be the only person on the floor. He would arrive to work every morning at 6:00 a.m. and maybe took 2 weeks of vacation a year.

While the CEOs certainly are not saying that you need to work 100 hours a week and never take vacations, they are saying that hard work will be a key factor in your success. So you need to develop a passion and a love for the work you're doing and for the people you're helping. Speaking to this, David Callecod (President and CEO, Lafayette General Medical Center) says that "I have always been told that you're a success when your avocation is your vocation. I really enjoy what I am doing and the challenges that healthcare presents everyday." Much like Gail Warden and David Callecod, if you enjoy what you're doing and are passionate about it, you'll never work a day in your life!

> " I find that the people who don't do as well as they should is because they are too caught up in process and not outcome. "

Determine the Key Outputs

As mentioned earlier, working smart involves determining the key outputs and ultimate goal of a project. Peter Karadjoff suggests that when someone asks you to do something, you should try and anticipate what they're looking for in the project: "Somebody will give you a set of instructions, because they want you to perform a specific job. You need to listen to them, do exactly what they said, and accomplish all the things as they narrowly defined them, but then think about where they are going with it and add a few more components." Peter made an effort to do this throughout his career. He would tell the person for whom he was doing the project, "Here is what you wanted, and, by the way, I was thinking about it and you probably would want to go this way as a next step." Peter would get responses such as "I was going to have to do that" or "I didn't think of that." He cautions that it's important first to ensure that you meet the minimum expectations and deliver on those before trying to anticipate what else someone might want. Wowing people involves competent follow-through, which is making sure that you cover the minimums, get the project done on time, and then anticipate where the person who assigned the project to you is trying to go with it. Peter explains,

> I have seen people miss the mark on this. Somebody will ask them for "X" and they will say to themselves, "I'm going to wow them and give them 'Y' instead." Unless you're really astute, you could really miss the mark. So make sure you cover the basics and then try to wow them.

Peter adds that even if it's a director or VP asking you for "X," you should ask yourself, "What does the CEO want?" Peter recommends that you think bigger than your current job and beyond what has been asked of you, and also think about the direction in which the CEO would want the project to go as well as what successes and impacts the CEO would deem most advantageous. Wearing the CEO hat when you're looking at a project will help you to put the tasks into perspective and make it easier to prioritize them.

Similar to Peter Karadjoff, Quint Studer says that it's critical for you to determine the key outputs of a project:

> You need to identify the desired outcome and make it as measurable an objective as possible. I find that the people who don't do as well as they should is because they are too caught up in process and not outcome. They think they've done something because they have worked hard or they figured out a process. But if you really want to separate yourself from the rest of the people, you need to know how to clarify with your boss

and others what the exact desired outcome is that they are looking for and then figure out a way to achieve it.

Determining the desired outcome and thinking bigger than your current job will allow you to "work smart" by prioritizing your tasks, determining the key outputs, and producing only the information that will provide the greatest results.

Focus on the Task at Hand

Working hard and smart also means focusing on the task at hand and not daydreaming about your next job or the job you wish you had. It means asking yourself every day, "What can I do today to create value for my organization and learn something new to move my career forward?"

Quint Studer recommends that you focus on your current job and quit worrying about your next one. He shared with me the story of when he was a vice president of a hospital and the COO position opened up. He got so caught up in thinking that he wanted to be the COO that he started doing a crummy job in his current position. Quint says, "Make sure that you do what's in front of you, and if you do what's in front of you and do a good job for the right reasons, the rest of it will take care of itself."

> Just do a great job and the work will speak for itself.

Peter Karadjoff adds that

> If you're doing something because you're using it as a stepping stone, don't worry if it doesn't turn out to be the stepping stone you thought it would be. Don't worry because I did this report and I didn't get the credit for it. Just do a great job and the work will speak for itself. So if you don't feel like you're getting credit, don't worry about it. You'll know, and it will be evident to others.

It was when Peter stopped trying to become a CEO that he became a CEO:

> I didn't worry about it. I wasn't worried about who was ahead of me or who was behind me, I just immersed myself in my work and I tried to be fulfilled with what I was doing. That is the most important thing, because at the end of the day being a CEO is just a job, and hopefully

you will have a family and other things. They might be proud of what you do, but they don't want you to spend more time at work.

———————————

The CEOs understood the importance of hard work and sacrifice throughout their careers, and these principles were critical to their success. So when you hear sayings such as "You reap what you sow," "A job worth doing is a job worth doing right," and "There is no substitute for hard work," don't roll your eyes. Rather, fully embrace the principle of working hard. Remember also that simply working hard or simply working smart will not alone lead to success. The combination of working hard *and* working smart will be the key to your success. Finally, remember the quote from Thomas Jefferson: "I'm a great believer in luck, and I find that that harder I work, the more I have of it." Don't allow the path of your career to be decided by others. Instead, work hard and work smart by making your experiences count, having passion for your work, and determining the key outputs, thereby creating your own luck.

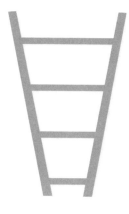

CLIMBING TOOLS

Work Hard and Work Smart

- Don't allow the path of your career to be decided by others. Instead, make your experiences count, have passion for your work, and determine the key outcomes.

- Success will come from the combination of working hard and working smart. And the difference between working hard and working smart lies in how you define and measure success.

- Don't simply work to work, but rather know what your end goal is and take on jobs that will function as stepping stones to achieving your career objectives.

- When you're working on a project for someone, wow them with the details, great follow-through, and by giving the person more than what he or she asked for.

- Think beyond your current job by thinking about the direction in which the CEO would want the project to go as well as what successes and impacts the CEO would deem most advantageous.

Climbing the Healthcare Management Ladder: Career Advice from the Top on How to Succeed,
by Jim Aldrich (Copyright © 2013, by Health Professors Press, Inc.)

- Ask yourself every day, What can I do *today* to create value for my organization and learn something new to move my career forward . . . and then do it!

Climbing the Healthcare Management Ladder: Career Advice from the Top on How to Succeed, by Jim Aldrich (Copyright © 2013, by Health Professors Press, Inc.)

4

Relationships Are Key

The CEOs recognized early in their careers that healthcare is a relationship-driven industry that requires a constant focus on creating, maintaining, and fostering relationships. Despite the CEOs having very different personalities and levels of charisma, they each went to great lengths to build strong relationships with their co-workers, subordinates, bosses, patients, physicians, board members, and countless others with whom they came in contact. They each said that establishing these relationships played a critical role in their success by allowing them to gain the trust and support of those around them.

According to American author and lecturer Dale Carnegie, "You can close more business in 2 months by becoming interested in other people than you can in 2 years by trying to get people interested in you." This really captures the importance of relationships and how taking the time to develop them will greatly benefit your career. The healthcare industry becomes more complex every day and, while having technical skills is important, your ability to build relationships, communicate effectively, and work as part of a team are what will ultimately determine your level of success. The key point that you need to understand is that unless you succeed in getting people to trust and follow you, all the technical skills in the world will not allow you to drive change and lead others. Theodore Roosevelt once said, "People don't care how much you know until they know how much you care." In other words, until people believe that you have their best interests in mind, they will not trust you to lead them. Each of the CEOs emphasized that successful leaders develop relationships, treat people with respect, and communicate in ways that foster, support, and strengthen relationships.

Working with Others

Due to the complexity of healthcare, no one person can be an expert in everything, and thus we must interact and work with others in caring for patients. It's often said that healthcare is an industry of "people taking care of people." I'd take that one step further and say that healthcare is an industry of "people working together to take care of people." Working successfully with others requires constant and effective communication and is a skill that needs to be developed and honed. According to the Center for Management and Organization Effectiveness, leaders and managers spend about 80% of their time engaged in some form of written or verbal communication.[8] In other words, as a manager you're not physically doing the work of caring for a patient; rather, you're communicating with, removing barriers for, and interacting with others to help them take care of people.

The act of communicating can be very complex, and even subtle changes in your tone of voice can cause others to misinterpret what you're saying. Thus you must take great care to ensure that others understand what you're saying and what your true intentions are. The following is a great explanation of the complexity of communication:

> A simple [hello] can transmit a lot of things. The voice's tone shows if the speaker is happy, pleased, bored, hurried, angry, sad, scared, aggressive, or dominant and the intensity of these states[:] irony, affection, support or joke.[9]

It's critical that your audience understands what you're communicating. Both your tone of voice and body language can greatly impact how your message is received. For these reasons, mastering the building of relationships and developing effective communication skills are prerequisites to your success.

Speaking to the importance of relationships, Jim FitzPatrick (Senior Vice President, Network Management and Development, Mercy Medical Center–Des Moines) received the best advice of his career from one of his bosses, who told him, "It's all about relationships, stupid!" Jim has experienced firsthand how absolutely true this is, that the people who flourish in the healthcare industry leverage relationships by being open and honest communicators, rather than creating wedges within the organization. He adds that, "Healthcare would be a really easy field to function in if we didn't have to deal with people, but we do, and it's a very important part of it." Jim suggests that those who don't develop an understanding of how critical relationships are should think about becoming a consultant—someone who can go into an organization, do his or her job, and then move on to the next client. A role such as this would allow someone to avoid having to deal with the emotional side of change and the people side of the business, and focus instead on contributing technical skills to an organization.

> " The most important skills to develop are your interpersonal skills in working with people and building trust in the organization. "

In this regard, Mike Slubowski prided himself when he was in graduate school, learning technical skills and concepts such as linear programming, decision trees, and discounted cash flows. He'd think about how he'd apply all of these skills in the real world and in the process create a lot of success for himself. Mike learned, however, that

> Leadership is way more about engaging and inspiring and dealing with the emotional side of change instead of simply the facts. You have to have facts, but you have to balance them with getting at the emotional side of change. So you really have to rely much more on your communication skills, your verbal skills, your writing skills, and your persuasiveness. Early on I really didn't understand the emotional side of change, but I came to appreciate it very quickly afterward.

Similarly, it wasn't until after graduate school that Rob Casalou realized just how important the people side of the business really is: "During graduate school you learn about marketing, finance, Medicare, and all kinds of other stuff, but when you get into the actual work environment, you find that 80% of what you're dealing with are people issues." As he climbed the healthcare ladder, Rob learned that the organizational behavior classes he took in graduate school were not about "touchy-feely stuff" and "just a bunch of fluff."

Kevin Unger has also been keenly aware of the importance of developing relationships and its impact on his career:

> I'm not the smartest guy around and I've never been very book smart. My grades were never real strong, but my ability to communicate and to get along with people has really paid dividends in my career. It was the people side of the business that has really been my strength and the reason for my success.

It's important to understand that while the technical skills you learn in graduate school are important and required for you to do your job well, it's the relationship skills you develop that will either make or break your career. Graduate schools realize this and have incorporated more and more group projects into their curricula. Peter Karadjoff notes that business schools require students to work in a lot of groups, and that at least half of the classes involve some type of group project. He recalls that,

> When I went to night school, I did a lot of group projects with other people who had full-time jobs. So you have a project to get done, you have 3 weeks to do it, and you have to work on it with four other people who also have full-time jobs. So to get the project done, you have to do it as a group and you have to figure out how to make it work.

At the time, Peter thought the intention was just to get the project done; looking back, however, he realized that this was probably the most real-life lesson that he learned in graduate school—how to facilitate groups to get things done.

Kevin Unger also stresses the importance of knowing how to work in groups or teams, because that is how hospitals are set up:

> Projects in school are team based and often times they can be a real pain because you may feel like you're having to pull or drag someone along and deal with all the dynamics involved. This is the reality of life and having a career in healthcare. So you need to embrace team projects and learn how to be successful together as opposed to just focusing on your individual grade.

We've all worked in groups, and most of the time you probably cringe whenever you hear a teacher or boss say "group project." Working in a team can be a challenge because there is usually no defined group leader, and thus the team consists of people who share no direct consequence for not following one another's lead. Speaking to this challenge, Quint Studer says that if you really want to get to the top or close to the top, then you can't always wait until people report to you to get them to do something: "You need to really understand that, to move your career, you're going to have to show that you can use various methods of leadership to align people to a goal, even when they don't work for you." When I asked Quint how you can get others who don't report to you to work for you to achieve a specific goal or outcome, he replied, "Make sure they know the outcome you're searching for and then try to help them figure out what's in it for them

> [A]s leaders we have to figure out how to explain things. If we don't, we lose the employees' belief in us.

or what's in it for the organization. You need to try to get them to agree to the plan and ask them if there are any barriers that would keep them from achieving the plan." Quint adds that you also need to provide reward and recognition to those individuals who help you. For example, if I worked on a team with Quint, he might send a letter to my boss saying, "I just want you to know that Jim Aldrich is on 'X' committee to get 'Y' done, and here's what he's doing to create real outcomes." "Make sure you're rewarding and recognizing people on the team," Quint says. "Don't get hung up on yourself getting the reward and recognition, because if people think you're doing it for your own recognition, then they won't do [the work]. But, if they know that by working with you, you can get them rewarded and recognized, then they will be more likely to do [the work]." Alternatively, if someone who doesn't report to you isn't cooperating or working with you, instead of saying "I notice that you're not doing something," ask "What can I do to provide better leadership to you so that you can be successful?" Quint says that most people will respond "You're doing fine" and correct their poor performance.

Because so much of the work done by healthcare executives is dealing with the human aspect of the business, Dr. Wayne Lerner (President and CEO, Holy Cross Hospital), who has an undergraduate degree in psychology, feels that executives are more like psychologists than anything else:

> People who are hospital CEOs are simply working as social psychologists, because they are people who work with other people on an indi-

vidual or group basis and are trying to get them to change their behavior in order to achieve the organization's goals. You can call it leadership or whatever you want, but it is simply social psychology.

You need to understand what it means to work in groups and with individuals. You must appreciate that people don't all have the same motivations, values, and interests that you do. In order to rise to the level of a CEO and eventually work with a board, you need to be involved in a lot of different situations, get a lot of different experiences, stub your toe a number of times, make some mistakes, and then learn and grow from them.

Similar to Wayne, David Callecod says that one of the skills that has made him successful in his career is his undergraduate training in speech. A speech major and a psychology minor in college, David says both degrees "have made me uniquely qualified to be an administrator. Just for the fact that so much of what I do is not only giving one-on-one interpersonal communication; but I am constantly giving 4 to 5 speeches a week to various groups. So the ability to communicate, the ability to structure an argument and to make a case, have been invaluable for me."

Building Trust

Developing strong relationships with others requires building a high level of trust with them. According to Kathleen Griffiths,

> The most important skills to develop are your interpersonal skills in working with people and building trust in the organization, because if you don't have that then you really can't get much else done. What has allowed me to be successful is the fact that I have developed solid working relationships and relationships with people who trust that I will do the right thing for the organization.

Rob Casalou adds that

> The thing that I appreciate the most about people and the people that I tend to promote and hire are those who seem authentic and genuine. They are not just trying to look good so they can be promoted, but rather they are down to earth, and when they screw up, they admit it and make good on it. They have a certain degree of humility and they are able to carry on a social conversation and build relationships. If you have those

qualities, then you will do fine, because these are the qualities that people gravitate to.

John MacLeod (President and CEO, Mercy Hospital) says that the best career advice he ever received was to be a servant leader:

> Servant leadership is what healthcare administration and hospital administration is all about. Many people see the CEO at the top of the organizational chart and think that everybody works for him/her. Technically that is true, but the really effective CEOs understand that they are servant leaders.

John says that he's flipped his hospital's organizational chart upside down, with patients and families at the top instead of the hospital board and CEO (Figure 4.1). As CEO, John sees himself as working for everyone else versus the other way around; his job is to give others the resources to do their jobs well for patients and their families and to get obstacles out of their way. He adds that

> You have to believe in people and that you work for them. They are the caregivers and they are the people who are on the frontlines laying hands on patients, while the administrators get to stay back in their nice, air-conditioned suites. Obviously there is a lot of pressure being a hospital CEO, but the bottom line is that the patients and the family see the nurses, doctors, and technicians and they don't see the CEO.

John believes that you'll be successful if you practice servant leadership throughout your career, because even as a frontline manager you need to serve the people who work for you.

When it comes to building trust and solid relationships, David Stark says that humor and being able to laugh at yourself are important qualities that make you more real and personable to others. "We deal with a lot of serious stuff, and it doesn't mean you have to tell jokes, but you've got to have a sense of humor," David says. He also stresses that having humility is important, and that this is especially true as you continue to move up the organizational ladder:

> The sooner you say you know it all or that you have all the answers or that you're the cat's meow, the sooner that you're going to get knocked down to size and your staff, physicians, and leadership team won't be there with you. Having a level of humility and servant leadership is important.

Figure 4.1   Mercy Hospital Cadillac Organizational Chart

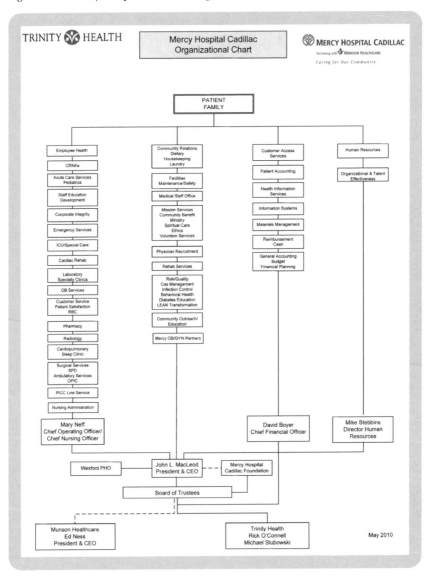

Dr. Wayne Lerner also agrees that having a sense of humor is important:

> In running meetings and working with people, you can diffuse a situation or make people feel at ease especially through self-deprecating humor, which can be a very valuable technique. You'll find people you work with that either have no sense of humor or use their humor at the expense of others, which is just not a good management style.

Wayne says that it's the human side of management that will allow you to become a great leader and achieve a significant level of success.

In addition to humor, being willing to step in and do whatever needs to be done will allow you to build solid relationships and credibility with others. David Fine shared how he learned this lesson firsthand while he was an administrative resident at the University of California Hospital in San Francisco:

> More or less my first day on the job, the CEO took me and the other resident on a tour of a new building that was scheduled to open soon to see at what stage of completion everything was and how much of a scramble there was going to have to be in the last few weeks to have it ready for the grand opening. When we got to the loading dock, the CEO turned to us and said, "Guys, tomorrow I want you to come here in jeans and I want you to clean this place up." I remember talking with my fellow administrative resident about how much we felt this really wasn't exactly why we had gone to graduate school. Later on in the course of my residency, which didn't include any other assignments like this, I talked to the CEO about the assignment he had given us that day. The CEO said that it was important in his experience to hire people for whom no job was too small and that you would be willing to do whatever was necessary to meet the needs of the organization.

This experience really resonated with David and he's adopted this trait in forging his career ascent, which has allowed him to build trust and strong relationships with others.

Communicating with Others

Developing relationships with others also involves being able to communicate effectively with them. Mike Slubowski says that often we incorrectly assume that when we communicate something to others that they're interpreting and understanding it exactly as we'd intended. He says that we all essentially have built-in filters due to our life experiences, level of education, and upbringing that can affect what parts of a conversation we hear and how we interpret what's said to us. Mike explains that

> It takes a lot of work, but you really need to understand how you need to communicate, how many ways you need to communicate, how many times you need to communicate, and how you can get people to engage and play back what they heard so you can understand whether or not they are getting your point.

An example of this comes from Kathleen Griffiths. In 2009, Chelsea Community Hospital was going through a significant merger with the St. Joseph Mercy Health System. Kathleen said that during the merger she felt as though she was talking about the process ad nauseam, but that she would still have people say to her, "Well, I never heard about that." "I would think, well, I've already talked about that 15 times," Kathleen says, "but I soon realized that you just can't overcommunicate, especially when you are going through [what] for Chelsea Hospital was a very significant change."

In addition to making sure that people understand what you're telling them and that you're telling them enough times, you also need to share with people your motivations. Quint Studer says, "We're normally good at explaining what needs to be done and how it needs to be done, but we don't take enough time to explain why." Quint shared the story of when he was talking with one of his employees at Studer Group, and the person said to him, "I really like working here because we don't talk about money, we just talk about making a difference." Quint saw the employee as feeling inspired and motivated to work for the group for this reason, which is exactly how he wants the group's employees to feel. Quint went on to say that Studer Group does well financially, but that is not why they do what they do. He tells his employees, "The reason we want to have new business is not to generate more revenue; it's so we can help more people." Of course, getting new business will generate more money for the company, but that is not the message that will get the employees fired up and excited to put in the work to contribute to the company.

Quint feels that most healthcare executives with whom his company works don't take enough time to explain the "whys," so people will *want* to do their job instead of thinking they *have* to do their job.

He gave the example of the nurse who asks "Why do you want me to bend over backward for this doctor?" Quint says that the leader's response should be, "We're not saying that you need to bend over backward for this doctor; but if we have everything ready for the doctor when he or she comes in, then the patient will get faster and better care. We're all about the patient getting better care, and if we're efficient, the doctor will be able to help more patients."

Quint adds that those at the top also have to help those they lead understand how doing something will benefit them. Doing this requires finding out what drives and motivates the person to do the job. He shared the story of when he was a hospital CEO and he had a group of people from another hospital come to learn about what his hospital staff was doing. One of the men from the visiting group broke away from the pack because he didn't want the programmed tour. He then approached a security guard and asked, "What do you think about what the hospital is doing to make it a better place for patients?" The guard replied, "I like it. From what I understand the more patients we have, the better job security I have, and right now I really need job security." Quint explains that the security guard figured out what his "why" or motivation was, and "for a nurse it might be eliminating a fall. I don't always know what that *why* is, but as leaders we have to figure out how to explain things. If we don't, we lose the employees' belief in us. And the key thing that leaders cannot afford to lose is people believing in their leadership."

In this regard, David Olson believes that "It's very important to get to know your staff and to let them get to know you. This builds trust, and trust is a two-way street. The best way to get people to believe in you is for you to believe in them."

> " The best way to get people to believe in you is for you to believe in them. "

He says that probably the best advice he's been given is to always work to make sure that everyone feels like they're in the "inner circle":

> Most of us have a close set of friends we talk to within our organization, but a successful leader expands his or her "close set of friends" to include people throughout the entire organization. Create an inner circle and enlarge that inner circle to include as many people as you can. This builds relationships within your organization and gives people the feeling that they can approach the President to get the straight scoop.

David went on to say that this isn't only true when you're a CEO, that you should try and create a large inner circle at all levels of your career. This is a very powerful way to manage people.

Similar to David Olson, Sean Williams says, "It is important to develop a reputation as someone who is honest, transparent, and not shy about acknowledging what you don't know." As a way to reassure and establish trust with others, Sean says that you need to say something along the lines of, "This is what I am trying to accomplish and this is how I think you can help."

Mike Slubowski wishes that he would have had a better appreciation early in his career of how change is technical, political, and cultural as it relates to explaining the "why." He says that most people tend to think about the technical aspects of change and that this is especially true for early careerists. Someone will launch an initiative to open a new clinic or put in a new information system and then tends to focus more on the project and tangibly getting it done versus also considering the political and cultural aspects of instituting change. Mike has learned that the political aspects of change, or who is being affected adversely or positively by the change, and the cultural aspects of change, or how change will affect "the way we do things around here," are as important, if not more important, than the technical change itself. He says that

> We usually underestimate the amount of time that we need to put into the political and cultural aspects of change, and they will submarine any change initiative. So you really need to spend two-thirds of your time on the political and cultural aspects of change. Additionally, this means that you can't do as many change initiatives, and you will have to pick your change initiatives very carefully and do them very well.

We tend to launch many projects thinking they're what we need to do and to just get them done, Mike says. The reality, however, is that you first have to engage the stakeholders and get their hearts and minds engaged in the change effort. You need to explain the "why" behind the change and create a burning platform for people, which will then allow them to become committed to the change.

Technical skills are helpful, but your real success will come from developing and fostering relationships with others. While this may sound easy, it isn't. According to renowned leadership and management author John Maxwell,

> Relationships are the glue that holds people together. They don't just happen automatically. We have to make deposits to develop and build relationships because relationships aren't forged out of accident. They are intentional and leaders understand the value of relationships because they know that leadership is influence and at the core of influencing other people is having good relationships with them. It's impossible to be a long-standing, continuing, successful leader that people willingly and voluntarily follow if you're not good at relationships. So learn to smile and always understand that relationships are the key to influence, which is the key to leadership.[10]

Developing solid working relationships will require work and a concerted effort on your part. Additionally, you will need to take time to make deposits into the emotional bank account of others and to really understand where they are coming from. Healthcare is a relationship-driven business, and establishing solid working relationships with everyone around you will be a critical key to your success. Regardless of what type of personality you have or your level of charisma, you can develop successful relationships by establishing trust and showing respect for others in how you communicate and relate to them.

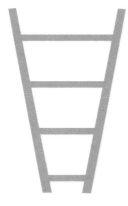

CLIMBING TOOLS
Relationships Are Key

- The field of healthcare requires a constant focus on creating, maintaining, and fostering relationships.

- All of the technical skills in the world will not allow you to drive change and lead others. People need to believe that you have their best interests in mind or they will not follow you as their leader.

- Your tone of voice and body language can greatly impact how your message is received by others.

- Don't assume that when you communicate something to others that they're interpreting and understanding it exactly as you'd intended. People have built-in filters due to their life experiences, level of education, and upbringing that can affect what parts of a conversation they hear and how they interpret what you are saying.

- Ensure that people understand what you're telling them and that you're telling them enough times.

- You need to explain the "why" behind a change and create a burning platform for people, which will then allow them to become committed to the change.

Climbing the Healthcare Management Ladder: Career Advice from the Top on How to Succeed, by Jim Aldrich (Copyright © 2013, by Health Professors Press, Inc.)

5

Variety Equals Success

The CEOs successfully climbed the healthcare ladder by gaining a variety of experiences both inside and outside their organizations. Healthcare is a complex and diverse industry and understanding the entire care continuum and how all of the pieces interrelate will be critical to your success. The CEOs emphasize the importance of developing an array of experiences throughout your career to continually enrich and broaden your understanding of all aspects of healthcare. They also caution that in most cases a single organization cannot provide all of the needed experiences, and thus you must look outside your organization for ways to gain insights. Reaching out beyond the walls of your organization will provide you with new environments in which to practice your skills and learn new ones. Looking back over their ascent to the top, the 29 CEOs also recognized the importance of not getting pigeonholed early in your career in a specific area. They continually looked for ways to diversify their experiences to help them grow and develop as healthcare leaders.

This principle differs slightly from jumping at new opportunities for the fact that, again, your single organization cannot provide you with all the diverse and varied experiences you'll need to be a well-rounded and successful executive. Your organization, for example, might have a different payer mix than another organization or might be in a rural setting while another might be located in an urban environment. The key point is that you can't expect or shouldn't even try to gain all the necessary experiences in one organization. This doesn't mean that you shouldn't work for one organization for your entire career; rather, even if one organization is giving you all the experiences you need, you should still look to other organizations to learn from their unique differences and challenges. You could, for example, attend a variety of professional conferences, network with people from other industries, or read a variety of professional journals. You need to reach out beyond your organization's walls and engage with people who might have a different mindset and set of experiences to see what new skills and insights you can add to your own toolbox and use to benefit your organization. A variety of experiences will bring perspective and clarity to situations and will provide you with frameworks from which to make decisions and drive successful change.

In this regard, Dr. Wayne Lerner says that his career success lies in the fact that he has not had what he would consider a typical career for a CEO: "If you look at the kinds of positions I've had, I've never managed professional departments like surgery or medicine, but rather I worked in the medical school with nurses and in the nursing college and with the support departments." By always being willing to jump in and take on whatever needed to be done, Wayne put himself in a position to be seen as the go-to person whenever anything came up and thus gained an array of experience. He shared the following story of how this approach has greatly benefited his career:

> One day my boss, Gail Warden, told me that he wanted me to take on a new assignment, I was going to transfer from Ambulatory Care to the Medical School, and that this would be a good experience. At first I was apprehensive and asked Gail how this move would affect me later down the road. Gail replied, "You don't even realize now how important this will become."

His boss was right; the experience proved invaluable because, from time to time, Wayne was asked to work as a consultant to assist other organizations with similar transitions. He also shared another experience of being asked by a community to assist them with developing a plan to build a rehabilitation center:

> I met with the leaders of the community, the Dean of the Medical School, the CEO of the teaching hospital, the head of one system, and the head of another system. By virtue of the fact that I have had such a varied career, I was able to speak directly to the issues confronting all of

them. Also, I appreciated the motivations of the people who are working with them. I was able to construct an agenda that created an opportunity for inclusion of everyone present. You can't do this if you've had a singular type of career. The deeper and the broader your experience base, the more comfortable you will be as you progress in your career.

When I asked Kevin Unger if he could go back in his career, would he do anything differently, he said, "No, I have had a broad range of experiences that all play in and contribute to being a CEO." When asked this same question, Denise Brooks-Williams (President and CEO, Henry Ford Wyandotte Hospital) replied that she wouldn't be where she is today if not for all of the different experiences she's had: "I feel that the good and the bad all contribute to who you are and where you are. I feel that the bumps in the road are what caused me to grow and then move on to the next level of leadership." Kevin and Denise make the point that certain experiences in your career may at the time seem difficult and like great trials, but that down the road when you look back on those experiences you'll see that they really helped to shape and refine you as a leader.

> " The deeper and the broader your experience base, the more comfortable you will be as you progress in your career. "

While having a variety of experiences in your career is important, it's even more essential to understand that you may need to be proactive in ensuring that you gain the necessary experiences. When I asked Rick O'Connell what he knows now that he wished he'd known when he first started his career, he said,

> You have to try not to get pigeonholed and you've got to try and have a breadth of experiences. What happens a lot today is that we find people who are up and comers and we put them in charge of "X," but then we've got to remember that we have to try and take them to the next level. So leaving somebody in "X" and just letting them thrive there if they truly have the ambition to be something more is something we have to watch out for. It is important to understand that not everybody wants to be a CEO and not everybody wants to be a COO, and if that is the case, then we need to find where they are comfortable as long as they continue to excel. But if they truly aspire to be something greater, then we need to help them along that career path by taking them out of a position and moving them into something else.

Rick adds that those climbing the healthcare ladder should be willing to move into a new area and to have that kind of dialogue with their boss, along the lines of the following: "Hey, if you're going to start a new product line or service line, I would love to get involved in that. Use my skillset any way you can. I would like to gain the new experience." You should not hesitate to express to your boss that you want opportunities to do more. Rick recommends asking to take on more even if an opportunity does not fall within your specific job description. Throughout his career he would be proactive in these ways, which allowed him to gain a variety of experiences and build a solid foundation in healthcare operations.

Similar to Rick O'Connell, Mike Slubowski says, "You need to take your career into your own hands, and you need to learn and reach out beyond the four walls of your organization." He adds that you can't expect that somebody is looking out for you and is mentoring you along the way: "If you find that kind of person, then great, and be sure to hang onto them. But if you don't, you will have to take some responsibility to reach out, network, and learn beyond your four walls." In addition to reaching out beyond your organization, Mike says that you can learn a lot about leadership from other industries and that you should not limit your experiences and discussions to those only within healthcare; rather, you should try and move out of the "healthcare box."

> You need to take your career into your own hands, and you need to learn and reach out beyond the four walls of your organization.

There will be times in your career when you'll need to be proactive in gaining new experiences and then there will be other times when new experiences will be thrust upon you. In either case, you'll need to be prepared to adjust and learn from any new experiences, good or bad. Each of the CEOs mentioned repeatedly that a healthcare career path does not follow a straight line, and that oftentimes the path will take many unexpected twists and turns. Nancy Schlichting's career was no exception. At one point she felt that she had been passed over for a promotion based on politics rather than performance. As a result, Nancy quit her job without having another one lined up and then took another job too quickly and decided that it wasn't the right job for her either: "So within a year I had changed jobs three times, and some people might say that it would just destroy my career to do this, but I didn't look at it that way." The experiences allowed her to step back and reassess her situation. Nancy subsequently took a big pay cut, returned to Akron, Ohio, and became the COO of Suma Health System with the hope that she would eventually succeed her mentor, Al Gilbert, as the CEO there. Nancy says, "It was a really good time for me and it was a healing time for me personally. It allowed me to gain my confidence back from the recent experiences I had." A year later Nancy received a call from Gail Warden asking her to come and work at Henry Ford Health System, which she accepted. Five years later, she became CEO of the entire system. She notes,

> You just don't know how things are going to turn out, and sometimes you have to do what's best for you personally and for your family, and sometimes you make the move that's best for you professionally, but your career is not going to be linear. It rarely is. And when you talk to most CEOs, they have gone through something in their lives that helped them rethink their situation. This is important to think about, especially when you're young and you think your career is going to be stepwise and it doesn't always work out that way.

It's important to understand that your career will take many turns, some of them good and some bad. You should always ask yourself what you can learn from each experience. In this regard, Dr. Wayne Lerner recommends that you ask yourself, from both a disciplinary and experiential basis, what are the kinds of experiences you want to have in your toolkit and how can you use one to build on another? For example, if you're involved in a United Way fundraising campaign for your organization, he says, "you should ask yourself, how does this experience teach me things about how I can be a better CEO?" Always consider what knowledge, skills, and insights you can gain from any situation or opportunity that will help you to become a better leader and executive.

You should also seek to gain new perspectives from people outside your organization. This approach greatly benefited Don Wegmiller in his career ascent. He always sought out groups and individuals outside his organization to learn from their experiences:

> I always tried to reach out beyond my own job and my own organization and interact with other people who were doing similar things, and I always learned an enormous amount from what they were doing—some of which was good and some of which was bad, some of which was applicable and some of which wasn't.

Don says that this sorting process is very helpful and that if you're only talking to people inside your hospital or health system, then you'll never become aware of what's going on in the rest of the field. He also shared his experience of having lunch once a month with a group of fellow residents:

> I was a resident in the Fairview organization in the Twin Cities, which had several administrative residents serving in hospitals throughout the Twin Cities. The residents all came from different programs and universities and they would get together and have lunch once a month. This lunch basically gave us a chance to find out what each other was doing, what we were finding, what we were learning, what's interesting, what's challenging, and what's different between our organizations.

Don learned a lot from these lunches and grew to understand that a great deal of his knowledge and experience was going to come from settings outside his organization: "Since I can't hold down jobs in three or four different organizations at the same time, how else am I going to gain these experiences?"

———————————

The key point that Don and the rest of the CEOs are making is that for you to be successful, you need to continually find ways to reach out beyond your organization and develop a variety of experiences. This approach will be critical to your success because job descriptions are usually narrowly defined and are written for you to complete specific tasks that the organization needs accomplished. They are not written with your personal career advancement and success in mind, and so you'll need to be proactive in reaching outside your job description and organization to learn from others and gain new skills. However you do it, ensure that you are exposed to people from many different organizations, and remember that variety equals success.

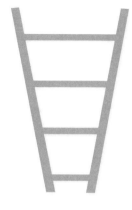

CLIMBING TOOLS
Variety Equals Success

- In most cases a single organization cannot provide all of the experiences you'll need to advance your career. Reaching out beyond the walls of your organization will provide you with new environments in which to practice your skills and learn new ones.

- Seek to gain a variety of experiences both inside and outside your organization, which will bring perspective and clarity to situations and will provide you with frameworks from which to make decisions and drive successful change.

- Always ask yourself what you can learn from each experience, whether good or bad.

- Determine the kinds of experiences you want to have in your toolkit and how can you use one experience to build on another.

Climbing the Healthcare Management Ladder: Career Advice from the Top on How to Succeed, by Jim Aldrich (Copyright © 2013, by Health Professors Press, Inc.)

6

Learn the Business

In addition to gaining a variety of experiences, all of the CEOs spent time on the front lines learning firsthand how their hospital and health system operate. The CEOs stress that to be successful you must gain a strong understanding of hospital operations and how all of the various departments and systems interrelate. While you do not need to have worked in every department or have a clinical background, you do need to have some exposure to the operations of various departments to gain an understanding of how decisions can affect different aspects of the hospital. The CEOs said that this in-depth knowledge only comes from spending time in the trenches and talking with the people who are on the frontlines every day carrying out the operations of the organization. No textbook or graduate course can give you a full appreciation of how complex hospital organizations are. The only way to understand the daily operations is to get in the middle of the action and see it with your own two eyes.

Speaking to the complexity of hospitals, renowned management expert Peter Drucker once said, "The hospital is altogether the most complex human organization ever devised." To put the magnitude of this statement into perspective, it's important to understand just who Peter Drucker was. His career spanned more than 6 decades as a writer, consultant, and teacher, and nearly 40 books discuss his ideas on management theory, practice, and policy for both business and nonprofit organizations. Drucker worked with many of the world's largest corporations; with small and entrepreneurial U.S. companies; with non-profits and agencies of the United States; and with the governments of Canada and Japan. President George W. Bush awarded Drucker the Presidential Medal of Freedom in July 2002 in recognition of his work in the field of management. Additionally, he received honorary doctorates from universities in the United States, Belgium, the former Czechoslovakia, Great Britain, Japan, Spain, and Switzerland.[11] I share all of this simply to make the point that Drucker's assertion that the hospital is the most complex organization ever devised is grounded in an entire career having studied businesses in numerous industries (he passed away in 2005 at the age of 95). To reiterate, you'll need to spend as much time as possible gaining experience and learning the fundamentals and complexities of a hospital organization.

Operations Experience

Consider that hospitals basically function as small cities and treat thousands of patients with hundreds of different diseases, ailments, and disorders every year. A typical 300-bed community hospital will discharge about 15,000 patients annually and perform procedures related to emergency services, cardiology, neurology, oncology, orthopedics, radiology, and nuclear medicine, to name a few. Furthermore, a hospital of this size remains open 24 hours a day, 7 days a week, employs about 1,400 staff members; and provides cafeteria, laundry, pharmacy, valet, and daycare services, among many others. At any given time, a hospital will house roughly 230 patients, who will stay for about 4 to 5 days and receive numerous visitors at all hours of the day. Additionally, the medical staff consists of about 600 to 700 physicians, all of whom expect efficient operations, timely results, and their patients to receive the best care possible. On top of all of this, hospitals must hold themselves to the highest quality standards and face regular inspections by city, state, and federal agencies to ensure that they're providing safe and appropriate care. Most people will need many years to fully understand how all of these aspects of a hospital must work together in a smooth and orchestrated fashion. Don Wegmiller says, "A hospital is

> You really need to understand the concepts of patient care and how care is delivered by working with nurses and physicians.

a very unique creature, and to simply go to graduate school and assume that you understand how a hospital or health system operates is, of course, a fallacy." He adds that one of his absolutes for people who want to run a hospital is that they first simply jump in and get a job in a hospital. Don says that it really doesn't make a difference what job it is; it can be as an orderly or a clerk in the billing office: "You simply need to get experience in the hospital setting and begin to understand how hospitals work, how physicians interact with hospitals, and what the operations are like at the ground level."

Jack Weiner says that people climbing the healthcare ladder will not be very successful without having an understanding of, for example, the clinical operations of a hospital. He compares the process of understanding how a hospital functions to learning the operations of an aircraft carrier:

> You can't understand the ship's problems if you haven't spent time in the boiler room, understanding where the pipes go, what it takes to clean filters, what a circuit breaker is, why they work, where the electrical panels run, and how the emergency power is structured. One does not expect to run an aircraft carrier without first understanding how the ship runs. That's why in the Navy you have to spend time as the ship Safety Officer, ship Engineering Officer, and perform other roles. You have to go through certain roles and responsibilities to fully understand how the ship operates. Running a hospital is a complicated operation, and you can't understand the problems of the medical staff and clinicians if you haven't spent time with them learning what they do.

Gail Warden offers similar advice:

> You really need to understand the concepts of patient care and how care is delivered by working with nurses and physicians. This will help you get a better understanding of what really happens on a patient care unit and in an ambulatory care center. You really have to understand the business if you want to be successful.

David Stark adds that

> You need to find ways to get exposure to the operations of the facility. Put on scrubs and go to the OR for a day, put on the environmental services uniform and clean a room, go to the dock and help unload a shipment, or go and sit in the ER for a Friday night. Go get that direct frontline experience to see what it's really like. This will be invaluable to you as you progress through an administrative career, and you will have an appreciation for how a hospital actually works.

Even as CEO, David continues to make it a point to get frontline experience from time to time, and says that anyone climbing their way up the healthcare ladder should do the same, not just up to when they become a CEO.

Speaking to the importance of actually doing the work, David Callecod says, "When you're young and you have a degree, you tend to go in and think that you can run things, but you've got to have a fundamental understanding of how each individual piece of the business works." Early in his career, David had the opportunity to work through the support side of the business. Every time he took over a new department he would actually go and work in that department for a day and learn what the staff did in dietary, pharmacy, housekeeping, and maintenance. David says, "I just think it's so critical to understand how all the pieces fit together as later on in your career you're making decisions. So I think that my ability to work up through the support side and to have been in the trenches has been invaluable to my success."

Dan Jones (former System Vice President, Ochsner Health System) says that the experiences he brings to the table that have contributed to his success are usually centered around building knowledge: "I assess the situation before I act on it or attempt to resolve the situation. It is a skill to be exercised, and the more experience you have on you the faster that comes." When he began his career, the first thing Dan learned was to do the job before you start to change or restructure anything. He adds that many people come in and assume that they know how a hospital operates; they don't take the time to learn the job, the politics, or the system. Dan spent the early part of his career pulling shifts in different jobs so he could learn exactly what people did in their different roles. He explained, for example, how he benefited from working a shift as a unit secretary, ER technician, and surgery technician:

> Doing this develops relationships and gives you perspective that you will never get from simply watching or hearing. The key to my success has been relationships, which pure and simply is being able to connect with people and respecting every role and every individual for what they provide and bring to the table. Understanding what goes on in the day-to-day operations and communicating the purpose for change, and not just making changes because it looks good on paper, is key to being a successful leader, and this is what engenders trust.

Developing experience working in the frontlines will help you make better, informed decisions as well as build relationships and credibility with frontline staff by showing them and others that you're willing to "roll up your sleeves and get dirty" to understand what the frontline staff is going through and experiencing.

While it's important to gain exposure to various areas of a hospital system by "volunteering for a day" and working with frontline staff, it's also essential to develop experience managing and leading departments that have operational components, such as Lab, Radiology, Rehabilitation, and Nuclear Medicine. When I asked Garry Faja how someone can develop these types of experiences, he said that from the beginning of his career he'd made it known that he wanted to gain operational experience. In 1979, Garry was working as a consultant on a long-range planning project for Oakwood Health System in southeastern Michigan. When the consulting engagement ended, Oakwood Health System offered Garry a job. He told them that he would take the job, but only if the position offered line operations experience, that he didn't want to come into the position solely as a planner. Garry says that this was an intentional decision on his part in that he didn't want to only go the direction of planning and be labeled as a planner: "I wanted to be labeled as an operator, and while this has probably changed in today's day and age, when I was coming up the ladder, once you got into the planning route, you would then be labeled as a planner and not as an operator."

> The key to my success has been relationships, which pure and simply is being able to connect with people.

When I asked Garry how someone can break out of a "planning" mold, he said: "You need to get some exposure to operations. If you're just a planner who only looks at market share data and you're not out there talking to people and seeing what their issues are, then you get stuck." Garry suggests that if you're a planner and want to get into operations, then you need to try and find ways to work with clinicians to understand their roles and issues. This is not to say that you should not go into strategic planning, because it's a skill that a healthcare executive must have and do well. Instead, Garry and the rest of the CEOs advise that you have some exposure to operations, because if you only work in planning or information technology or performance improvement or human resources, then you might not be getting enough exposure to the overall fundamentals of how a hospital generates revenue.

It's important to note that while several of the CEOs came up through the strategic planning side of the business, they were not working as planners 100% of the time. Rather, they found ways to make sure they were also involved in the operations side of the business. For example, Jack Weiner held the title of Vice President of Planning, Marketing, and Business Development at Foot Memorial Hospital for 7 years. In addition to holding this title, he was also an associate administrator and directed the operations of the ancillary, professional, and support departments. Nancy Schlichting worked as assistant director of operations for 1 year and then as associate director of planning for 2 years. She had some operations experience and thus was able to subsequently become the COO of Akron City Hospital after 2 years of planning experience.

> You don't go to school and then start your career. You're constantly learning something.

When I asked Peter Karadjoff if there were any areas that those climbing the healthcare ladder should avoid working in, he said, "It is tough to say, because if you do a good job in any realm, you can be successful and will get noticed." He says that whatever the job is, just immerse yourself in it and do the best you can:

> You might be completely flexible to turn everything down and not get pigeonholed, but most people aren't. Most people at some point, particularly after they finish their fellowship, need to find a job that has health insurance and can pay their bills. So you're going to have to take the human resources job or the IT job or the supply chain job, even if you think it might pigeonhole you. Just jump in and wow everybody.

Dave Spivey adds that

> You need to get involved in projects and initiatives that will expose you to the broader aspects and components of the organization. If you do this, then opportunities are going to emerge out of projects that you work on and you will have a more broad-based perspective.

It's important to understand that you never know which projects, initiatives, or committees you get involved in will open doors for you down the road. By understanding as many aspects of the organization as you can, you increase your value to the organization and, as a result, put yourself in a position to be given new and challenging assignments. Dave explains that, "It's not a bad thing if you go down a specific career track, but you need to make sure that whatever track it is, it will be able to give you exposure to the broader aspects of the organization and doesn't get you pigeonholed."

The key points are that you need to develop operations experience and to be mindful not to pigeonhole yourself. In some cases you may not have any control in this regard and you'll need to simply do the best you can with any opportunity you're given. You should still, however, try and find ways to gain exposure to the operations of your hospital or hospital system, whether by volunteering for projects that provide clinical exposure, talking with physicians, or shadowing clinicians.

Clinical Experience

While the clinical side is where the hospital makes its money, Jack Weiner says you don't need to have a clinical background to be successful in running a hospital:

> For those of you who have an MHSA or an MBA and do not have a clinical background, you need to go and work with the clinicians and understand what their issues are. If you can understand how all the pieces work, then you can understand the clinicians. You need to find projects that have clinical inputs and clinical activities, where you work directly with clinicians and understand what they think, how they think, and what their issues are.

Jack's point is that you can't be successful if you don't understand what clinicians do and what their needs are.

While clinical experience is not a must for you to be successful, it's certainly beneficial if you have it. Betty Noyes spent many years as a nurse and thinks that the experience of working directly with patients has been invaluable in her career growth: "I knew what it was like to not have a suction machine when you need one, I knew what it is like to not have cooperation from other departments across the hospital. I knew what it was like to work three shifts in one week and what it is like to work every place from the newborn nursery to the ICU in the same week. I could bring a sense of experience and therefore credibility with the nursing staff since I rose up in the ranks of nursing."

Betty recommends that people who are not nurses and who have no experience working directly with patients need to gain some type of clinical experience through an internship or by shadowing someone who is at the bedsides. Betty adds that she's not biased toward nursing and that the experience could be in respiratory or physical therapy or the like, "but you need somebody to give you that perspective of what this business is all about." As an example of the importance of gaining clinical experience, when Betty was the vice president of nursing at Georgia Baptist in Atlanta, she would have every MHA intern shadow her for a week or two. She would then send them out to the nursing unit and tell them "go pick and go do." Betty says that

> One of them went on to become a CEO, and he and I still laugh about the whole experience, because he remembers the joys and sorrows on the unit and they got to see everything. They saw me banging my head against the wall, as well as being on stage. So my advice for anybody that is striving to succeed in healthcare is that you've got to get some experience touching base with the patient.

In addition to gaining clinical experience, working your way up from the front lines of an organization and not advancing too fast will allow you to have time to really learn and understand the operations. Bob Milewski says that, "The best executives in terms of solid, long-standing careers work their way up through the chain of command and they learned and added to their career over time." He describes this knowledge base as taking shape during the formative early years of a career and as coming from working different shifts and learning about scheduling people, budgets, overtime, and supervising others:

> As a pharmacist, I worked nights, weekends, and all kinds of different shifts. I was a supervisor and I scheduled people as I went up the ranks. Even to this day, when people start talking about things like problems with HR and discipline issues or the various HR systems, I know what they are talking about and it's really helpful. It is helpful for me, but it's also helpful for them, because they know that I know what they are going through and it builds credibility.

Bob thinks it's important to take jobs working in the lower levels and then slowly moving your way up the ladder. One of the worst career failures he has seen was when he promoted someone who was an extremely talented person and who had just finished an MBA program. Bob said that they were having a tough time finding a department administrator and so they put a recent graduate in the position because the person understood the division and had been in the organization for a few years. In the end, however, he says the person failed miserably

> because they hadn't worked their way up through the chain of command and hadn't learned the needed supervisory skills. Somebody jumping up too fast and too many steps in their career can be very dangerous to

their career. So it's better to work your way up through the ladder even though it takes time and is frustrating. Your career will move along fairly quickly if you're talented.

As you gain new experiences and learn the frontline operations of a hospital, you also need to recognize when it's time to "let go" of certain tasks so you can take on new ones. Garry Faja explains that

> The stuff you did to be successful early in your career is not the stuff that is going to make you successful later in your career. You've got to learn and take on more, but then let stuff go. Maybe when you first started out you did a lot of work as an analyst and that was a lot of detail work and a lot of analytics, but as a CEO you're not going to do that. You did it and you know how to do it, but you need to let go of it because you can't climb the ladder if you don't let go of the previous rung.

As you advance up the healthcare ladder you will need to begin to focus on overall strategy and the big picture of the organization, rather than just on the details at the ground level.

Keep in mind that the learning process is continuous as you advance through your career; you'll need to be a lifelong learner. As Peter Karadjoff explains, "You don't go to school and then start your career. You don't go from learning to doing. You're constantly learning something. So don't think that you've stopped your learning process." As he looks back on his career, Peter says that he learned how a hospital runs while he was a management engineer, he learned how a doctor's office functions while he was managing practices, he learned about solving institutional problems when he served as the "operational improvement guy" for Trinity Health, and he has learned about the medical staff and new aspects of hospital operations in his role as a CEO. "You're always learning," Peter says, "so make sure that you keep that hat on and understand that you're never 'there.'"

It will take you many years to fully understand all of the complexities of a hospital organization. But don't get overwhelmed. Just jump in and begin "learning the business" one day at a time.

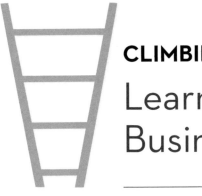

CLIMBING TOOLS
Learn the Business

- Learn how your hospital or health system functions by spending time in the trenches talking with the people who are on the frontlines carrying out the daily operations of the organization.

- Developing operational experience will help you make better decisions by understanding how all of the various departments and systems interrelate, will give you credibility with staff, and will increase your value to the organization, thereby putting you in an advantageous position to be given new and challenging assignments.

- Find projects that will allow you to work directly with clinicians to understand what they think, how they think, and what their issues are.

- Recognize that as you advance up the healthcare ladder you will need to focus more and more on overall strategy and the big picture of the organization, rather than just on the details at the ground level.

Climbing the Healthcare Management Ladder: Career Advice from the Top on How to Succeed, by Jim Aldrich (Copyright © 2013, by Health Professors Press, Inc.)

SECTION 2

Managing Your Career

Having learned the key success factors employed by the CEOs and now having a foundational knowledge of what it takes to be successful, this next section will discuss the critical importance of understanding that these habits, actions, and skills alone will not ensure your success. While these traits will allow you to be productive, knowledgeable, and seen as a "star" at work, without the proper career management, the success factors alone won't allow you to achieve all of your career goals. Each of the CEOs also went to great lengths to carefully manage their careers in terms of being vocal about their goals, deciding when to transition to another position or organization, choosing whether to work in a small or large hospital, and leveraging their experiences to avoid being pigeonholed into one role or area of expertise.

The concept of managing your career is similar to the role that an agent performs for a professional athlete. The agent's primary role is to think about the big picture and to help guide and direct a client's career. Not having an agent could result in the athlete getting stuck playing for a bad team, a team that doesn't effectively use the player's skills, or a team that fails to recognize his or her full potential. The same is true for your career: without a conscientious and concerted effort on your part to manage each stage of your career progression, you could get stuck working for an organization that doesn't utilize your talents, fails to provide you with opportunities to grow, and only succeeds in taking you further away from your goals.

Since healthcare executives don't typically have agents thinking about and managing their every career move, you'll need to be your own agent. You know that you have the skills, talent, and desire to do the job, but now you have to make sure others know that as well. As you read this section, continually ask yourself, "Am I being an effective agent for myself and, if not, what more could I be doing?" A world-class professional athlete wouldn't settle for anything less than the best, and neither should you!

7

Being Vocal

As a highly-motivated person climbing the healthcare ladder, a big dilemma you'll face is finding a balance between being vocal about your career goals and being overly vocal to the extent that people perceive you as disingenuous or self-indulgent. This can be difficult to do since we've been taught that business and career management is all about "survival of the fittest," "the squeaky wheel gets the oil," and the louder and more persistent you are, the more attention you'll get from the boss. So how do you find balance and avoid crossing that fine line?

To better understand how the CEOs managed this dilemma, I asked them the following questions:

> What was your mindset moving up the ladder, and how vocal were you about your career goals?

> How vocal should people today be about their goals and aspirations?

> When should someone make or not make their career goals known?

With every interview I completed, it quickly became clear that when it comes to being vocal about your career goals, the answer is not simply black or white, but rather a hazy shade of gray. All of the CEOs agreed that being vocal is good for your career and certainly needed, but they also cautioned that it really depends on your particular situation, with whom you're speaking, and what your organization's culture is in regard to career development. Despite these words of caution, all of the CEOs suggested that the benefits of being vocal certainly outweigh the potential negatives.

Let It Be Known

Kevin Unger recalls that,

> I was never shy about what my goals were, and that I wanted to work toward having the necessary background to one day be a CEO. I was pretty up front about it so people could give me advice and mentor me and give me their input on how to achieve that.

Phil McCorkle offers similar advice, saying that people need to take it upon themselves to ensure that they're getting the experiences they want and need and then letting people know if they aren't. Phil adds that most people are not going to ask you, "Hey, Jim, what do you ultimately want to be or what would you like to do next?" Rather, you need to give your supervisor a signal that you really want to do "X" or that you would like to get experience in "Y." Phil explains,

> You really have to take the initiative and be deliberate about making what you want to do known, and then asking for opportunities. You just have to at least ask, and in today's world you've got to be a go-getter. It's a lot more competitive, and so you need to be real deliberate about where you want to be and have a road map of where you'd like to go.

Rob Casalou adds that while it's important to be vocal, it's just as important to be specific:

> It helps to be as precise as possible with the organization as to what you want to do. A CEO can't read your mind and so you shouldn't ask a question like, "What do you think I should do?," or say something like, "I really want to be considered for any opportunities." These are too open-ended and don't provide a clear direction to others of what you want to do.

Rob recommends that you say something such as, "Here are the areas that really interest me, and I would like to be considered for 'X' role."

Providing this level of specificity about which areas and positions you're interested in will allow others to begin to slot you into a certain career track, and when a spot opens up, they'll be more likely to recall the interest that you expressed and consider you a good fit.

Keep in mind that even if you don't get the specific job you originally asked for, making your interests known will cause others to think of you whenever a similar position opens up in the future. For example, you may say to your boss that you'd like to be the service line leader for oncology someday. While that job may not currently be available, a position as the service line leader for cardiology may open up and suddenly your name is on the list of potential candidates simply because you made it known that you're interested in taking on that type of position. The key point to remember is that specific questions get specific answers, and specific requests get specific results. If you give your boss a general request such as "I'd like to be considered for any opportunities," then the best response your boss can give you is, "Well, I'll keep you in mind if anything opens up." Contrast

> You really have to take the initiative and be deliberate about making what you want to do known and then asking for opportunities.

this with a specific request to your boss: "I'd like to be the service line leader for oncology someday. What do I need to do to prepare myself for that type of position?" Making specific requests and asking specific questions will allow your boss to respond in a specific way, such as, "Well the current leader has been in that position for about 3 years and will probably be taking on a new role in about 6 months. I'd be happy to consider you as a candidate for that position, and in the meantime why don't you try to complete a project in the cancer center or take a class in budget management." Your specific request will allow your boss to understand exactly what you'd like to be doing as well as allow him or her to advise you on what you can do to become a strong candidate for the position. Furthermore, during that 6-month period your boss may be more likely to observe your performance a bit more closely and ask him- or herself from time to time, "Would Jim be a good fit for that position?" This is beneficial because, rather than having a one-time interview like other future candidates, you'd have 6 months to work hard and show your boss that you have what it takes to do the job.

Will It Be Well Received?

In addition to being vocal and specific about your career goals, it's important that you put yourself in a position in which this type of conversation will be well received. For example, if you're performing poorly in your current job, then trying to engage your boss in a discussion about your long-term career goals will fall on deaf ears. Additionally, your boss will probably scoff at the idea of helping you achieve higher levels of responsibility when you can't even handle the ones you currently have.

Speaking to this point, Quint Studer says that when it comes to being vocal about your career goals, you first need to understand what's expected of you (goals) and what success looks like (results). He recommends that you say something along the lines of the following to your boss: "One year from now I want to exceed your expectations. Tell me exactly what I need to accomplish to exceed your expectations." Once you've clarified what the goals are, then you need to deliver the expected results.

Once you've achieved the expected results and demonstrated that you have the ability to handle higher levels of responsibility, then it's appropriate to engage your boss in a conversation about your career goals. Quint suggests initiating the discussion by telling your boss, "I am very much committed to my own professional development, and I would like to ask you a few questions for my own growth."

These questions include the following:

What do you feel I do well, because I want to make sure that I continue to perform in a manner that produces results and is beneficial to the organization.

In which areas do I excel and which tools and techniques could I improve?

What training and development do you recommend for me right now to improve my skillset?

Do you feel my priorities are specific enough and well focused, and am I taking on the right responsibilities and projects?

Quint says that in being absolutely honest with the person about where you want to go, you also need to welcome his or her feedback and direction. It's important to ask your boss if your priorities are correct because priorities change; you might be working on something that you think is a big priority only to find out that it's no longer the big priority you thought it was. Quint also recommends that you check in periodically with your boss regarding your priorities to ensure you're on the right path to achieving success in the areas that are important to your boss and the organization.

Jack Weiner advises that you shouldn't be vocal about your career goals simply for the sake of being vocal. First, achieve some level of measurable success and then make your desire known that you want to move to the next level. Furthermore, the only way to know exactly what your boss considers success and great results is to ask for specifics and then deliver on those expectations.

> "[T]he best way to prepare yourself for your next position is to be successful in the one you're in."

While talking with your immediate boss is important, it's also beneficial to share your career goals with other people both inside and outside your organization. When it comes to speaking with people who are not your boss about your career development, Peter Karadjoff recommends that you pay attention to how you frame the conversation:

> When you're trying to network with somebody and you simply cold call them and say, "I would like to get to know you and network a little bit and see what opportunities you have there." If you frame the conversation in this way, generally you are less likely to get accepted and they are less inclined to give you their time. The same is true in your organization. If you go to one of the VP's and say, "I'd like to talk to you about a job." What does that person think? "Well, I don't have anything to offer, so I don't really want to talk to them."

The advice Peter gives is that you not frame the discussion around "networking" or "finding a job"; rather, you should tell the person that you'd appreciate his or her advice and that you'd like to learn more about what led to his or her success:

> People love to talk about themselves and are really open to these types of conversations. They will even create time when they didn't have it, if you naturally start a dialogue and genuinely ask for some advice. Additionally, these types of conversations will get the person's wheels spinning and they may say, "Oh, you like to do that? I didn't know that about you. I've got a friend who is doing that or we were just thinking about doing that."

Peter says that these types of conversations are more likely to influence the person to brainstorm potential opportunities for you. This approach will also prevent the conversation from feeling one-sided and as though you're only there to see what the person can do for you. Framing the conversation as a genuine back-and-forth mentoring dialogue will open doors for you and alert others to your career goals without having you seem disingenuous or self-indulgent.

Success Begets Success

While being vocal and specific about your career goals will help ensure that you're moving in the right direction, there's no substitute for hard work and achieving success in your current role. In other words, "success begets success," and if you're successful in handling your current responsibilities, then further responsibilities will be given to you.

The biggest problem Jack Weiner sees with people who are just finishing graduate school is that they're asking themselves, "What's my role and how do I get to the next level?" "What they don't understand," Jack says, "is that whatever role they are given is the stepping stone to the next level. If you want the next level, make yourself absolutely invaluable to me and blow me away with everything you're doing, and then I can't afford to not give you the next level." When someone comes into his office and asks, "When do I get to go to the next level?," Jack tells them, "Show me the results of what you have done."

> I find many people attempt to manage their career based on time frames rather than experience.

A perfect example of working hard in your current position and getting results is Sean Williams, who had a rapid ascent up the career ladder, becoming a CEO at the age of 33. When I asked Sean what led to his success and how vocal he was about his career goals, he said that he was fortunate to have worked for some outstanding executives who gave him great advice. One of these executives was John Sheehan at St. Luke's Hospital in Cedar Rapids. According to Sean,

> John is very focused and understands how to get things done. I will never forget the advice he gave me, which was that the best way to prepare yourself for your next position is to be successful in the one you're in. This really spoke volumes to me, because your track record should speak for itself. If you find yourself having to trip over yourself reading your

résumé to someone to convince them that you're really good at what you do, then maybe you're really not.

Sean says that what really helped him to climb the ladder was succeeding at each level by doing what needed to be done. He explains that, in essence, he didn't specifically say, "This is what I want to do and this is where I want to go." Rather, he expected that when he was successful in any role, that either his current employer or a potential future employer would recognize his efforts and would then give him additional opportunities to learn, grow, contribute, and succeed.

Similar to Sean Williams, Dan Jones was not vocal with his mentors, supervisors, or peers about what he wanted to be doing. Instead, he focused on doing the best job possible for the people he supported:

> I have learned that the people who try and manage their career are typically the ones that tend to fail and fall short. It is important that everyone have a career plan and exercise that plan; however, I find many people attempt to manage their career based on time frames rather than experience. You cannot successfully run a marathon without exercise and practice. It's those that focus on doing the best they can in the role they have today are the ones that eventually succeed. What people fail to recognize is that everybody is watching, regardless of whether you feel that or not, and those that attempt to manage their career and position themselves based on the wrong variable are the ones that stumble and fail. Whereas, the ones that focus on the product and the service are the ones that ultimately succeed and move up the career ladder.

While the advice from Sean and Dan may at first seem contradictory to what the other CEOs advised earlier in being vocal and specific about your career goals, they all emphasize the need to first achieve success in your current role before voicing your career goals to others. Going back to the example of the athlete and his agent, it would be very hard for even the best agent in the business to negotiate a lucrative contract for an athlete who is viewed as being a poor performer and not willing to work hard. The same is true in your career; you need to first establish who you are on the "playing field" or in your work environment and then let your actions and successes speak for themselves.

Yes, but . . .

At the beginning of this chapter I noted that when it comes to being vocal about your career goals there's a gray area that comes into play depending on your particular situation, with whom you're speaking, and what your organization's culture is regarding career development. You'll need to assess your unique situation and then proceed accordingly.

Speaking to this, Carrie Owen Plietz says,

> I think you have to be very aware of your surroundings and who you're talking to. You need to read the situation correctly, but you do need to be vocal and up front about the experiences you want to have, how you want to step out of your comfort zone, and how you want to grow. Otherwise you might miss out on opportunities right in front of you just because you didn't step forward and say that's what you wanted.

This advice captures the feelings of all of the CEOs. While being vocal is important, you first need to conduct an assessment of your specific situation, which means you'll need to take into account many different aspects of your career development and ask yourself the following types of questions:

Have I been successful enough in my current position to warrant having a conversation with my boss about my career development?

Do I have a clear idea of where I want my career to go and what next step I want to take?

If I discuss my career development with my boss, will I accept and welcome feedback, even if it's negative?

Will my boss feel threatened if I bring up a discussion about my career development?

If my boss isn't open to discussing my career development, then whom else can I speak with inside or outside the organization?

Are the particular questions I have better answered by someone outside the organization to avoid a potential misunderstanding?

After you've carefully considered these types of questions, then you should have a clearer idea of what you want to accomplish, with whom you should speak, and how to frame the conversation.

Once you've assessed your situation, Don Wegmiller advises that you keep your goals to yourself or only share them with friends or associates outside your current organization:

Inside your current organization, discussions about your personal career have as much opportunity to be misunderstood as they are helpful. If you're comfortable that your boss is a career-developer type, then that might be one person inside your organization to share your goals with. Even then, however, it's fraught with the potential for misunderstanding.

Don gives the example of a boss thinking to him- or herself: "This person obviously is very articulate about wanting to be a CEO. But I don't think he's going to be a CEO at this organization, so why don't I cut him loose at a future opportunity." He explains that,

> Well, that may be good for you and it may come exactly at the wrong time. This could be good since you're not wasting your time in an organization where you're not going to advance, but alternatively you may not have any other job opportunities at the moment, and being let go from your current job could be the last thing you need. So having these discussions with people outside that you trust, who aren't going to misunderstand it because they are not in a position to do anything about it, except to help, encourage, and mentor you, is the better option.

Don benefited greatly during his career progression by having job-related discussions with one of his classmates and close personal friends from graduate school, Scott Parker, who used to be the CEO of Intermountain Healthcare. He and Scott would share their experiences all the time, and since they both worked for different health systems their discussions were personal and confidential. Again, however, Don cautions that

> Had I been having those same conversations inside my organization, they would have been misunderstood. So I think that it is important to have those thoughts, discussions, and plans, but it's also important to be mindful of who you have those conversations with, and you need to pick those people very carefully. So the simple answer is yes, but with whom, when, in what detail, and why are all important questions to answer before just saying "yes" and telling anybody about it.

Similar to Don Wegmiller, Bob Milewski also recommends carefully choosing with whom to share your career goals. He recalls a piece of advice from Zig Ziglar, businessman and motivational speaker, who said that you should share your "go up" goals only with those people who love and care about you and your "give up" goals with everybody else. Bob explains that

Basically you're giving up smoking, you're giving up eating sweets, and you're telling everybody this because they are going to help keep you accountable. But sharing your "go up" goals about where you want to go and what you want to achieve, you have to be very careful and share these with a mentor, a friend, or a spouse. I have discussed this principle with many people that have personally experienced that when you share personal goals it is a very competitive world and human nature is such that people don't want you to be successful. They don't want you to achieve things that they haven't, and they try to discourage you. So you need to be very careful in sharing your "go up" goals and aspirations with other people.

To Be Vocal or Not To Be Vocal: That Is the Question

"To be or not to be: that is the question." In the play, Hamlet is making the comparison between the pain of life, which he sees as inevitable, and the fear of the uncertainty of death. Hamlet is dissatisfied with his life, but he can't be sure of what death has in store.[12] While being vocal about your career goals is not as dramatic as Hamlet's question, it can be equally as scary. So when deciding when and when not to be vocal about your career goals, it's important that you first make sure that you're successful in your current role. Then assess your situation to decide whether a conversation with your boss about your career development would be well received at the current time. Finally, be specific with your boss about what you want to do and achieve, and remember that "specific requests" get "specific results." Note that if you really think that entering into an open dialogue about your career goals is not going to be welcomed or that your boss will in some way try to sabotage you, then you're probably in the wrong organization anyway.

It's critical to understand that to move your career forward you'll need to be willing to do your own self-promotion and be your own cheerleader. At the same time you need to avoid being too vocal in promoting yourself, especially if you're failing to achieve success in your current role. The answer to the question "To be vocal or not to be vocal?" will change from time to time throughout your career. Sometimes the answer will be to be a little more vocal or to say nothing and simply work a little harder. Either way, as you tiptoe this fine line, be sure to continually ask yourself, "Am I being an effective agent for myself and, if not, what more could I be doing?"

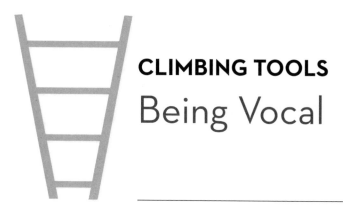

CLIMBING TOOLS

Being Vocal

- Take the initiative and be deliberate about making your career goals known and asking for opportunities.

- Achieve some level of measurable success before engaging your boss in a discussion about your career development.

- While talking with your immediate boss is important, it's also beneficial to share your career goals with other people both inside and outside your organization.

- Be as specific as possible when discussing with your boss what you want to do and what you would like to achieve. Knowing which areas and positions you're interested in will allow others to begin to slot you into a certain career track.

- There's no substitute for hard work and achieving success in your current role. If you're successful with your current responsibilities, then additional ones will be given to you.

Climbing the Healthcare Management Ladder: Career Advice from the Top on How to Succeed, by Jim Aldrich (Copyright © 2013, by Health Professors Press, Inc.)

8

Managing Career Transitions

Throughout your career you'll be faced many times with the decision of "Do I stay or do I go?" The answer to this question is usually, "it depends"—on how long you've been in your current position, what additional experiences you want to gain, which organization the new position is with, does it pay more money, will the move bring you closer to friends and family, and the list goes on and on. At some points in your career the decision to stay or go may come very easy; more commonly, however, the best decision will not be an obvious one. Numerous external factors can cloud your decision to take even the most promising of jobs, such as not wanting to move your kids into a new school or move away from elderly parents or cause your spouse to leave his or her dream job just so that you can chase yours.

In addition to these external factors, the decision to stay or go can be fraught with potential unintended consequences. For example, changing jobs too often may lead to being labeled a "job hopper," or as someone who's more interested in career advancement than the organization's goals. Additionally, a change in jobs might earn you more money in the short term, but could result in getting pigeonholed in one area and actually slowing down your career growth. In contrast, deciding not to accept a job offer may signal to others that you're content with the status quo and aren't looking for bigger and better opportunities, when the complete opposite is true. The key point is that your decision to stay or go is one that can have a significant and long-lasting impact on your career.

To better understand how the CEOs managed these decisions throughout their careers, I asked the following questions:

How do you know when it's time to move on?

How do you pick the best job for you?

Is it better to stay with one organization or work in different organizations to gain new perspectives?

While deciding whether to stay or go can be difficult and while your choice can vary at different times in your career, understanding the answers to these questions will greatly assist you in making the best decision for your specific situation.

How Do You Know When It's Time to Move On?

We've all heard the expression "timing is everything," and we've all probably benefited from good timing at some point in our lives. While fortune and luck do play a role in good timing, they should not be relied on when it comes to managing career transitions. For this reason it's important that you assess your level of passion for the work you're doing, your ability to learn and grow in your current role, and how well your values align with your organization. Conducting an honest and critical self-assessment of these key factors will help you to achieve good timing.

Not Passionate about the Work

It's important to have passion for the work you're doing. Once that's gone, you should think about moving on. When I asked Dan Jones how he knew it was time to move on, he said,

> You begin to develop a sense of flatness. It's almost like when you leave a Coke with the top off and after a while it gets flat. The same is true with your career when you begin to say, "Geez, this is the fifth or sixth time I've done this." The first couple of times were interesting, but it's not interesting anymore and it's just plain flat out not fun. When you've done your umpteenth annual budget, the next one really isn't quite so interesting anymore.

Dan adds that once you've run out of fresh ideas and the energy to take a group or team to the next level, then you need to think about moving on:

A lot of people don't recognize this early enough and it really comes down to are you excited when you get out of bed in the morning and can't wait to get to work. As long as you have that feeling, then you should have the energy and creativity to keep moving the team forward in your current role.

Similarly, Quint Studer says that it's time to move on when you've already achieved your targeted outcomes. Going forward you'll probably only be able to achieve incremental outcomes and they are not the ones that will really

> " It's time to move on when you've already achieved your targeted outcomes. "

excite you. "When you feel this way, it's time to move on," Quint says, "but you may not be able to move on, and this can be a great thing because this means that you have to look at how you can grow yourself in your current job."

The main point that Dan Jones and Quint Studer are making is that people who are passionate about their jobs tend to be happier, work harder, and achieve more success. So once you've lost the passion and sense of excitement for your current role, then you need to begin looking for other opportunities that will stimulate you and bring out your full potential. Additionally, it's important to note that just because you realize it's time for a change, new and exciting opportunities won't just magically appear. You may have to look for a while to find the right next job, and in the interim you should try and find ways to continue to "grow yourself" in your current job. This could include volunteering to be on various committees, getting involved in professional organizations, or looking for ways to take on additional tasks and assignments that nobody else wants to do or has the time to do. Carrie Owen Plietz really drives this point home:

> Being a healthcare administrator is hard enough, and if you don't love what you're doing, then there must be something else out there you would really love to do. We spend the majority of our life at work, so don't waste your life at a place that you don't enjoy because there is always something better out there.

So the first key question to ask yourself is "How passionate am I about the work I'm currently doing?" This question comes first because regardless of how much you're learning and growing and how well you like your boss and your organization, unless you're passionate about what you're doing, you'll never be happy.

No Longer Learning and Growing

The second key factor alerting you that it's time to move on is when you're no longer learning new things and growing your skillset in your current position. Denise Brooks-Williams says that she tries to go into every new role with a plan and will ask herself the following types of questions:

> Why am I taking this role?
>
> Will this role allow me to develop a skill that I'm lacking?
>
> Am I taking this role to determine if I like this area?

Denise adds that

> You need to go into the role with some goals of what you're trying to learn, and one way you will know it's time to transition is when you've learned what you decided you needed to learn when you first took the job. If you went into the job because you wanted to assess if you like it, then it might be a little more superfluous to decide when it needs to end. But for me, career transitions have been a little more natural because I can almost feel when its time to move on because I've accomplished all that I set out to accomplish.

Similarly, Garry Faja says that he didn't want to stay stuck in a job where it was just the same old job: "As long as people were giving me more opportunities to learn and grow, then I was perfectly happy." As long as you have this kind of learn-and-grow philosophy, you'll find yourself moving up the ladder. Garry notes that "As long as I kept getting increased responsibility, then I was perfectly happy. But if I wasn't, then I would move."

Phil McCorkle says it's time to move on when you're enjoying your job the most and you're at your peak:

> You want to walk away from the job when everybody is going to feel really disappointed that you're leaving and when you have added some successes to your résumé. It is all about achievements and what you have done for the organization lately. Don't get to a point where you become stale or you haven't done anything for a year.

He adds that, "If you're not going to be able to do it or if they're not going to allow you to do it or give you the opportunity, well then you've got to get out of there."

Phil makes the point that your career and tenure in your current position can have peaks and valleys. When you take on a new job you normally hit the ground running and look for new ways to make changes and add value, but then once you've achieved some early successes it becomes easier to grow complacent and rely on the early successes to carry you to the next level. Sometimes, however, the next level doesn't come right away, in which case you can't say, "Three years ago I successfully implemented 'X' process and cut costs for 'Y' department." You need to continue to learn and grow, and if your current organization isn't giving you the opportunities to do so, then you need to think about moving on before you allow too much time to pass without really accomplishing anything significant.

When starting a new position, Denise Brooks-Williams says that along with a plan for what you want to learn and what new skills you want to acquire, you should also know what results you want to accomplish and how they'll help you in eventually moving on to your next role. She explains that for leaders and managers the work is always going to be there. For example, if you manage customer service to the top decile, it's very likely that those results will eventually come back down again. So somebody is going to have to come behind you and manage it back up to the top decile. Or when you finally achieve top decile results, what continues to challenge you? During the course of her career, Denise says, "I haven't focused so much on just the issues in front of me that might always be there, such as I am going to fix 10 things and then I can move on. If you have that as your goal, then you would never progress, because the organization's cycle of change will always create new challenges." She adds that you create your next opportunity by accomplishing things, and so you need to go into a position knowing what the low-hanging fruit are and what are the results that you want to accomplish so you can then move to the next level and make the greatest impact. Setting learning and achievement goals will help you to know when it's time to move on.

> "Setting learning and achievement goals will help you to know when it's time to move on."

Don't Share Values with the Boss or Organization

When your personal values do not align with those of your boss or the organization, then you know it's time move on. This may come to light with a change in leadership or a recent merger. Whatever the case, once you and your boss can no longer see eye to eye and you no longer support the organization's mission, you need to think about moving on.

Speaking to this, Alan Channing says that

> Sometimes the decision to move is in your control and sometimes it is not. If you are in a position and the organization around you is changing because of new leadership above you, then that may be a time to look for new opportunities either in the organization or outside the organization.

Rob Casalou adds that

> It isn't all about money and sometimes you quit your boss and not your job, because you don't share values with the person you're working for. In contrast, you may share the values and like everybody, but professionally you do not feel stimulated by the job anymore.

Money, title, and prestige are not enough to sustain you. Organizations are continually changing, and often these changes are out of your control. Unless you're willing to adapt and change as well, you could be left behind. Also, not all change is good. A new boss may have different plans for your career and may even change the strategic direction of the organization. Both scenarios can play significant roles in your decision to stay or go.

In addition to not sharing values with your boss, you may just get to a point where you've hit the ceiling in your organization and you've advanced as far as you're going to go. Gail Warden says that

> You know it's time to move on when you're hitting your head on the ceiling. When I worked at Rush Presbyterian Hospital, I reached a point where I had a lot of conflict with the CEO because I had my own ideas and had been around long enough to know what I thought needed to be done versus what the CEO thought needed to be done.

Gail notes that this happens to a lot of people, and that "This is when they then need to find something else since they are not going to be able to accomplish much more than what they have already accomplished."

So when you're trying to decide the right time to move on, be sure to conduct an assessment of your current level of passion for the work you're doing, your ability to learn and grow, and how well your values align with the organization to increase your chances of achieving good timing.

How to Pick the Best Job for You

Realizing that it's time to move on is only the first step in managing your career. You also need to make sure that the next step you decide to take will provide you with new growth and learning opportunities and not just simply be the same role in a new organization.

Dan Jones says that when you're not being given new responsibilities or your current job isn't challenging you enough and you begin to think about what your next job will be, you need to know what challenges and opportunities your next job would need to have for you to decide to move on. He notes that

> A lot of people will just trade one set of not-very-interesting-challenges for another set of not-very-interesting challenges. So it's one thing to understand when the time is right and it's another to understand what it is that you want to move to. Moving from one CEO position to another might be very good but, on the other hand, a year later, it might be the same stuff that you were doing before and it's just in a different town.

Dan has found that people have a pretty good idea as to when it's time to go, but they don't have a very good idea of what they want to do next. He'll ask someone, "Why are you taking that job?," and the person will say, "I want to do something different." And then when he asks what that is, the response is, "I don't know yet, but I think I'll know it when I see it." Dan says that

> I don't buy it that you will know it when you see it, and by that time it's too late. You may have already taken the job and it may or may not be what you thought it was. So planning, investigating, studying, and talking with other people are important to knowing when it's time to leave and where to go.

Tom Priselac sums up this approach by noting, "You need to constantly be asking yourself what is the next experience that I could have, that would help broaden my knowledge base and my expertise?" Betty Noyes truly put this mindset and strategy into practice as she developed her career by always asking herself, "What is it that I haven't done?" She recalls that

> I would sit back and say, well, Mount Zion was a 670-bed teaching hospital that was connected with the University of San Francisco, and they had interns and residents from every type of medical and social services

school. So I had done that. So what else do I want to do? Well, I always wanted to work for a consulting firm because I wanted to see the world. Ok, did that. What else do I really want to do? Well, I have never been the Dean of a School of Nursing, so I will pursue that.

Betty would proceed down this line of thinking whenever she started feeling as though it was time to move on. Each new position she took allowed her to gain new skills and add to her knowledge base:

> I then took a position as a CNO, which also involved overseeing a 3-year school of nursing. So now I had that experience under my belt, which then led me to Herman Hospital, where I had a huge span of control with many different people, nine ICUs, and I opened new programs. Additionally, I had oversight for a licensed practical school of nursing, which I could keep under my wing because I had had the other previous experiences. I then said, "What do I want to do now?" Well, I haven't been in a multi-hospital system, and so I found Community Hospitals of Central California and was able get that corporate experience.

Eventually Betty was recruited by a for-profit health system to be the CEO of one of the new hospitals they were building, which allowed her to have a chance to build a hospital from the ground up. After meeting her husband, Betty decided to open her own consulting practice to have a more flexible schedule. The example she sets is that you need to know what you haven't yet experienced or accomplished in your career and then be willing to go and give it a try. Rather than just simply taking a new job for the sake of taking a new job, you need to determine what new skills the position will add to your toolkit and how they'll build upon your previous experiences.

> "[M]ost people don't take enough time to consider what is the best organization for them."

Similar to Betty Noyes, Kevin Unger would also take a step back and assess what types of experiences he hadn't yet had in his career. When he was hired as the VP of Planning and Strategic Development at Poudre Valley at the system level, and then decided to take a position in a hospital as the VP of Operations, Kevin says, "To some people this could be considered either a lateral move or even a demotion within the health system, but I did this just to get the operations experience in order to become a CEO at some point."

In addition to knowing what new experiences you want to gain, you should also have a strong sense of whether the culture of the new organization you're thinking of working in aligns with your values and core beliefs. Speaking to this, Garry Faja says:

> One of the things that people climbing the ladder need to know is how to select the organization that you want to work for. For most people, and especially new graduates, it's all about find a job, find a job, find a job, rather than finding a job that best fits them. Even though any job is good experience, most people don't take enough time to consider what is the best organization for them.

Garry recommends that you ask your potential new employer the following types of questions:

What kind of exposure will I get to the medical staff?

Will I have opportunities to sit in on governance meetings?

Will I be able to be part of a team working on X?

What is your management philosophy?

You should also ask yourself the following:

Am I a good fit with this organization?

Do they tend to be inclusive?

Do they enjoy their work?

Do they find humor in what they do?

Garry notes that these are the important questions to ask yourself because challenges and problems tend to be the same, no matter what organization you work for. It's the people for whom and with whom you'll be working who are key considerations when selecting your next job. In this regard, Garry took a job as a management consultant right out of graduate school and had the opportunity to work in many different hospitals throughout Michigan:

> I always liked St. Joe's in Ann Arbor and I thought that if I could ever work for any hospitals in Michigan, and there were only a few that I would consider working for, that one of them would be St. Joe's. So when the job came up at St. Joe's, I jumped on it. It wasn't just the next job, rather I knew a little bit about the organization and that it would be a good fit for me.

Even if you know what new skills you want to gain and whether or not the organization will be a good fit for you, your decision may still not be an easy one to make. Mike Slubowski says that to help him with these types of decisions he'll create a "T" account and list the potential advantages and disadvantages. Additionally, he will write out his thought process to better weigh the advantages and disadvantages. Mike notes that

> Early careerists are usually less bound by family considerations, and these decisions get more difficult as you get farther into your career and get married and have children. Also, different factors weight differently over time for you when making your decision. At the end of the day you really just have to trust your gut and you have a sense that you have accomplished everything that you think you can accomplish given the circumstances, and then you have to evaluate the strength of a given new opportunity.

Now that you know it's time to move on to the next job and what the best next job is for you, you also need to decide if that next job should be inside or outside your current organization. Although you may have already thoroughly assessed your current situation, this decision still requires some thoughtful consideration.

Staying in One Organization for a Long Period of Time?

When I asked Rob Casalou, who had spent 20 years with the Providence Health System, if it's beneficial to work in a variety of organizations, he said, "There is probably some value in moving around without becoming a job hopper, because it would give you a variety of experiences." The reason he didn't leave Providence wasn't because of a lack of opportunities to do so, but because his career was on such a trajectory that Rob was consistently being given new experiences and was able to go from a student intern to CEO in only 10 years. Rob said, "Every time I was thinking about leaving, another opportunity came up." For example, he was planning to leave Providence for another CEO position when he was then given the opportunity to build a new hospital, and so he decided to stay. Rob notes that

> You can create multiple experiences within one organization. I was at Providence for 20 years, but it sure didn't feel that way because I was in Southfield facility for 10 years and then in Novi facility, and the work was night and day. Additionally, we went through multiple mergers and so I felt like I had worked in 4 or 5 different organizations.

What kept Rob at Providence for so long was that constant sense of renewal.

Phil McCorkle spent 25 years with Butterworth Hospital in Grand Rapids, Michigan. He did everything imaginable in the hospital during that time and eventually became the CEO. When he finally left the organization, search firms would tell him that he did a poor job at managing his career by staying in only one organization for such a long period of time. Phil recalls that

> Even though I had gone all the way from an Assistant Director to CEO in one organization, they still said that I did a poor job. But, every time I would go and look at another position in another organization, I would come back to Butterworth Hospital and think nothing compares to Butterworth. It's a fantastic place.

While staying in one organization for a long period of time ultimately benefited Rob Casalou and Phil McCorkle, their experiences are certainly the exception to the rule. More often than not one organization cannot provide you the array of experiences you'll need to grow your career. You may need to be willing to move to a new city or state to find the job that best meets your desired next career step, even if that means moving away from friends and family. Speaking to the possibility of having to move, David Olson says that

> When you're first out of school and you're young, single, have no kids, and no obligations, that is the time you can be more flexible in your moves. Once you have other responsibilities, so much more thought must go into that next career move. For example, I just made a career move in the past 6 months. I was at Bay Area Medical Center for 11 years, and I loved that job and could envision myself being there forever. I had the job down, the board was very good, and we were growing, but I had to make a decision about managing my career. I recognized that I hadn't yet worked in a large metropolitan market. I had worked in Cedar Rapids, Iowa, home to roughly a quarter of a million people, but that was a long time ago, and we live in this world of "what have you done lately?" My last 10 years of experience had been in a more rural market in a community of only 35,000 people and in a completely independent hospital.

The other big piece of David's initial decision not to move was that he was really committed to staying in Wisconsin because all of his family lived there. He told recruiters, "It's not that I don't want to move, it's just I only want to move if it's the right thing." David's recruiter friends would tell him there are so few opportunities and that to limit himself both geographically and by type of the organization is like looking for a needle in a haystack in trying to work out the next career step. David took this advice to heart and decided he really needed to change his frame of mind. So when the position of President of Columbia St. Mary's in Milwaukee became available, he thought it would be a good opportunity for him because it would offer the big city experience he had been missing and would be very important in his career development: "I knew that I had to make a move, and while I was comfortable in my previous job, I knew that being uncomfortable sometimes is part of managing your career, and that making this move was an important stepping stone I needed to take."

As you try to decide "Do I stay or do I go?" step back and assess your current job situation and recognize that your decision can have a significant and long-lasting impact on your career. Take the time to ask yourself, "Is now the right time to move on? What is the next best job for me? Should my next job be inside or outside the organization?" Managing your career transitions effectively will not only help you successfully climb the healthcare ladder, but will also allow you to enjoy the ascent.

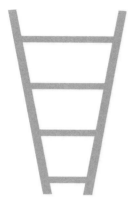

CLIMBING TOOLS
Managing Career Transitions

- When deciding whether to stay in your current position or to move on to another, first assess your level of passion for the work you're doing, your ability to learn and grow in your current role, and how well your values align with the organization. Conducting an honest and critical assessment of these key factors will help you to achieve good timing in managing your career transitions.

- When planning a career transition, know what challenges and opportunities your next job would need to have for you to decide to move on and what results you want to accomplish. You should also have a strong sense of whether the culture of the new organization you're thinking of working in aligns with your values and core beliefs.

- Carefully consider whether your next job should be inside or outside your current organization. More often than not one organization cannot give you the array of opportunities and experiences you'll need to grow your career.

Climbing the Healthcare Management Ladder: Career Advice from the Top on How to Succeed, by Jim Aldrich (Copyright © 2013, by Health Professors Press, Inc.)

- It may take a while for you to find the "right" next job, and so in the interim it's important that you try and find ways to continue to grow your skillsets and create opportunities for yourself in your current position.

- Continually ask yourself, "What haven't I experienced or accomplished yet in my career?" and then go and try it. Determine what new skills the new position will add to your toolkit and how they'll build upon your previous experiences.

Climbing the Healthcare Management Ladder: Career Advice from the Top on How to Succeed, by Jim Aldrich (Copyright © 2013, by Health Professors Press, Inc.)

9

Big versus Small Hospitals

Yet another dilemma faced by those climbing the healthcare ladder is whether to work in a large or small organization. While this decision may seem trivial on the surface, in reality it can have a very significant impact on the course of your career and the types of experiences you'll be exposed to. As a result, this decision should not be taken lightly and will require you to conduct an in-depth assessment of your personal and professional career goals.

The reason that this is such an important decision is because hospitals come in many different shapes and sizes and treat dramatically different types of patients depending on their size, type, and location. According to the American Hospital Association, in 2010 there were approximately 5,754 hospitals in the United States (Table 9.1).[13] While all of these organizations essentially have the same mission, vision, and values, they nevertheless vary greatly in terms of the types of populations they serve, the treatments and services they offer, and the number of employees they require to operate. They can range in size and scope from a 25-bed critical access hospital (CAH), such as Kenmare Community Hospital in North Dakota, to a 1,270-bed academic medical center, such as the Cleveland Clinic in Ohio, which treats every disease known to man using the most advanced medical technologies.

While, in general, an organization of one size is not necessarily better than another, depending on your personal career goals and the

Table 9.1.   U.S. Hospital Types and Locations (2010)

Hospital type	
Total number of U.S. registered hospitals	**5,754**
U.S. community hospitals:	4,985
nonprofit community hospitals	2,904
investor-owned (for profit) community hospitals	1,013
state and local government community hospitals	1,068
Federal government hospitals	213
Nonfederal psychiatric hospitals	435
Nonfederal long-term care hospitals	111
Hospital units of institutions (prison hospitals, college infirmaries, etc.)	10

Hospital location	
Number of community hospitals in rural areas	1,987
Number of community hospitals in urban areas	2,998

experiences you want to obtain, an organization of one size may in fact be better for you personally. A small hospital, for example, can provide you with an opportunity to wear many different hats and manage a variety of departments. It can also allow you to be a big fish in a small pond and gain a broad exposure to all aspects of the organization. While this might be good experience, small organizations tend to be viewed as less complex than larger ones. Even though you may have effectively managed a lot of different departments, your ability to handle a larger organization may be called into question.

> [I]n smaller places it is often easier to see how you make a difference and it's easier to develop relationships.

Alternatively, a large hospital can provide you with an opportunity to work in an organization that functions like a small city, where you could manage a large number of people and operate within a complicated organizational structure. While this may also be considered good experience, due to the significant complexities in such a large organization, you'll be given a narrow scope of influence and will have to work for many years before reaching the senior leadership level. The key point to understand is that both types of organizations will provide you with great learning opportunities and experiences, but depending on which one you choose, you'll need to take a different approach when it comes to managing your career.

To understand how the CEOs effectively managed this decision, I asked the following questions:

> What are the advantages and disadvantages of working in a small versus a large hospital?

> How can someone most effectively leverage their experience having worked in either size organization?

The decision is ultimately up to you as to what is the best size organization, and will depend on your own personal and professional career goals.

Bigger Isn't Better

Speaking to the advantages of working in a small hospital, Kathleen Griffiths says that

> First of all, you get to wear a lot of different hats and you do a lot of different things because you just have to in a small hospital. You don't have the resources, so we all get involved in a lot of different things. Also, I think that in smaller places it is often easier to see how you make a difference and it's easier to develop relationships.

There were a couple of times in Kathleen's career when she had some opportunities to work in a bigger place, but she has always really liked being in a small facility such as Chelsea Community Hospital (113 beds). Kathleen adds that

> I have found when I talk with colleagues who have worked in a big place that they tended to be more siloed, whereas my knowledge base may have been broader. Perhaps not real deep, but it was just broader by nature of being in a smaller place and doing more things.

David Callecod started his career in a small hospital with 120 beds and he thought it was perfect because he was able to learn how the whole hospital worked:

When you're at a big institution, like an academic medical center, it's pretty hard to learn anything more than what is going on in your own department, because once healthcare gets that complex, there's a lot of knowledge that goes into it. So I think that in a small hospital you're able to more readily see the whole picture.

> There is a difference in the complexity of managing a small facility versus a big facility.

David tells the people he mentors that if they can be a CEO in a 40-bed hospital or an assistant administrator in a 400-bed hospital, then he thinks early on in their careers it would be much better for them to go and work in a smaller facility. In a smaller facility you would have an opportunity to gain an understanding of how the entire organization operates and be the person who is ultimately responsible for its success or failure. This experience is invaluable, and if you're able to get it early in your career, it will provide you with a great foundation to continue to grow your leadership competencies.

An example of this is Sean Williams, who at the age of 33 became the CEO of Jones Regional Medical Center, a 25-bed CAH in Anamosa, Iowa. Sean says, "It wasn't by some grand design that I started my career in a small hospital, but now when I look back I'm very glad I did." Sean notes that as a CEO in a small hospital it is very clear what you are responsible for—all of it. He notices that for his colleagues who work in larger hospitals at the VP level, sometimes it can become unclear as to where their responsibilities begin, where they end, and how much direct control they have. Sean explains that,

> For example, they may be responsible for a given department, but the success or failure of that department may be directly influenced by another department that they don't have very much interaction with or very much influence over. Whereas in a smaller hospital setting, you traditionally have a lot of autonomy, and in a CAH you're kind of it. So the plus side is if things go well, you get a nice pat on the back, and if things go poorly, even if it's beyond your control, you get to answer for it. The pressure that comes with that prepares you for what it means to truly be in a leadership role, where the accountability for good and for ill really ends with you, as it should.

Jim FitzPatrick also took the top job at a smaller hospital. He took a fellowship position after graduate school and, midway through, the organization began laying off people, and so Jim began to investigate other opportunities: "My dad had a connection for a job at one of the local hospitals to be an associate director for quality, and I even thought about going into the military to do hospital administration, but I then learned about an opportunity to be the CEO of a small rural hospital that was a part of a Catholic health system in North Central Iowa." He had two mentors at the time and told both of them about his options and asked what they thought he should do: "Both of my mentors said that if you go rural you will never regret it and you will get to experience and touch a lot of stuff. You will be the jack of all trades, and so I was advised to take the rural opportunity." Jim learned that the assistant director for quality position was a staff role in which he would run a lot of reports for people and wouldn't get to carry a project through to fruition. So at the age of 24, he decided to take the CEO position and run Eldora Regional Medical Center, which was a 25-bed CAH in Eldora Iowa.

Jim emphasizes that he would not have taken the job if the hospital had not been a part of a larger health system:

> I am too much of a believer in systems and the resources that you can have as part of a system. Eldora Regional Medical Center was part of a health system and so if I didn't have something, I knew that I could always call the "big house" where they had Master's-prepared Human Resources people, a pharmacist with a Ph.D., and the surgical expertise that I never would have the resources to afford. So I recommend working in a small hospital as long as it's part of a larger system.

Similar to Jim FitzPatrick, when I asked Rob Casalou which size organization is better for someone to work in, he said,

> There is no better. It really depends on the work environment and the kind of organization that you want to work in, and it might depend on what is available. If you have a choice, you should pick a hospital that is a part of a system because it is hard to go from a stand-alone tiny hospital and then leap into a larger one.

It Comes at a Cost

While a small hospital can provide you with a broad exposure to the entire organization, a sense of being close to the patient, and clear lines of authority, these aspects can come at a cost. Kathleen Griffiths says that some disadvantages of working in a smaller hospital are that you don't have all of the resources a bigger place has, you may not have the stimulation from a larger group of colleagues with broader experience, and there isn't much opportunity for advancement. To this latter point, Kathleen notes the lack of turnover in the higher ranks at her hospital:

> At Chelsea Community Hospital we don't tend to have a lot of turnover. Our Chief Operating Officer has been here for 35 years, our Chief Human Resource Officer has been here for 30 years, and our Chief Financial Officer has been here for about 19 years. This is always a limitation of a small organization, and when you have real talented stars in your organization, it's often difficult to find places for them to go and so you risk losing them.

In addition to not having many opportunities to move around in a small organization, Sean Williams says that you'll have limited resources and may end up in a scenario where no matter how good you are, you may not be able to succeed as an organization, and this failure will reflect on you. Sean adds, "There can also be a perception outside the CAH world that it's easy to manage because of your cost-based reimbursement. Additionally, the margins can be tight and recruitment to rural areas is challenging."

In addition to the lack of adequate resources and managing razor thin margins, David Stark says that

> The longer you spend in a critical access hospital, the harder it will be to move to a bigger facility, because you will be pigeonholed. There will be the issue that, yes, you can handle that, but I don't think you can handle a bigger organization. You can go from big to small throughout your whole career, and it's a lot easier because you can say I've done this and that, and it's assumed you can handle a smaller facility. While in a small facility you may have an opportunity to do a broader range of things, there are a lot fewer managerial responsibilities at a 25-bed CAH than there are in our four-hospital system in an urban market.

In a large organization, the medical staff can have five or six competing groups, three different primary care organizations, and a staff of 1,000 physicians. Whereas at a CAH they have a staff of maybe 12 doctors who all rotate who will be the president of the medical staff. So you know all of them and you probably play golf with them also.

David said that while it may still not be easy to govern the medical staff at a small facility, it is much easier than putting together a management agreement with a group of orthopedic surgeons, understanding the differences between the interests of the vascular surgeons and the cardiothoracic physicians, and how that dynamic works with three different emergency departments and different levels of subspecialty. He says,

> It's harder to learn this, because you've been so used to a fairly simple structure where you can actually get around and communicate with the whole medical staff. It's very difficult to communicate to 1,000 physicians, and from this standpoint there is a difference in the complexity of managing a small facility versus a big facility.

Further clarifying the differences in complexity between large and small facilities, Jack Weiner says that a governing board of a 350-bed hospital looking to hire a new CEO would be more likely to hire the COO of a 500-bed hospital than the CEO of a 100-bed hospital:

> There is an assumption that in the larger hospital they have had to deal with more complex issues, have had broader medical staff involvement, and are better suited to deal with the complexities in a 350-bed hospital. This is not necessarily true, but when I look back at the steps to become the COO of a larger hospital, it is more complex than if they came from a small one. I have a lot of respect for the CEOs of smaller hospitals, because they do everything I do and they know everything I know, but they do not have the support staff that I have.

In the end, the decision whether to work in a small or large organization really comes down to where you want live, what your ultimate career goals are, and what experiences you want to obtain. If your goal is one day to run an academic medical center, then you would benefit from getting a job in one and then working your way up. If you prefer instead the idea of being a big fish in a small pond and are willing to live in a rural area, then you should pursue that opportunity, as long as the hospital is a part of a larger health system. Or you could choose to work in a medium-sized hospital and have the best of both worlds. The key point to remember is that there are about 5,700 hospitals in the United States and, regardless of which one you work in, you will need to manage your career and continually find ways to grow your skillset.

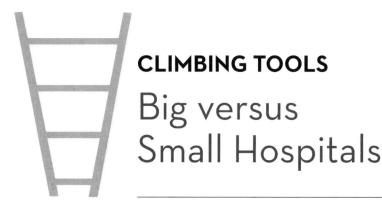

CLIMBING TOOLS

Big versus Small Hospitals

- No one size organization is better; your decision whether to work in a large or small hospital setting or system will ultimately depend on your personal career goals and the experiences you want to develop.

- Working in a small hospital will allow you to gain a broad exposure to all aspects of how the entire organization operates and to develop leadership skills in being the person who is ultimately responsible for its success or failure.

- If you decide to work in a small hospital, choose one that is part of a larger health system so that you can tap into the resources (human and capital) of the broader system.

- The potential disadvantages of working in a small hospital include limited resources in comparison to a larger organization, not as many opportunities for advancement, and difficulty in trying to transition to working for a large hospital (small hospitals are generally viewed as less complex than larger organizations).

Climbing the Healthcare Management Ladder: Career Advice from the Top on How to Succeed, by Jim Aldrich (Copyright © 2013, by Health Professors Press, Inc.)

- Working in a large hospital will allow you to operate within a complicated organizational structure and provide you with an opportunity to manage a large number of people.

- The potential disadvantages of working in a large hospital include having a narrow scope of influence due to the complexities of an organization of its size as well as having to work for many years before reaching the senior leadership level.

Climbing the Healthcare Management Ladder: Career Advice from the Top on How to Succeed, by Jim Aldrich (Copyright © 2013, by Health Professors Press, Inc.)

10

Leveraging Your Experience

As the field of healthcare becomes more complex and as increasingly more pressure is placed on organizations to provide high-quality and safe care, those climbing the management ladder are being given narrower roles with a limited scope of influence. Gone are the days when an early careerist could move from administrative fellow to assistant administrator to vice president and then to CEO in an 8- to 10-year span. The field has become far too complex, and developing a full understanding of all aspects of healthcare will take many years. This means you'll need to carefully choose which area you want to focus on first, knowing that regardless of which you choose you'll continually need to leverage the experiences you develop to transition into other areas that will expand your skillsets and move your career forward.

The areas most often chosen by individuals coming out of graduate programs or fellowships have been process improvement, physician practice management, or consulting. These have become the popular choices by virtue of the fact that the industry demands it and, thus, these are the areas where the jobs are. Healthcare organizations are being asked to do more with less, and organizations without a competency in process improvement and Lean Six Sigma thinking and methods are not going to survive. Additionally, healthcare reform is incentivizing hospitals to lower their number of admissions and re-admissions and, therefore, ambulatory and physician practice management will continue to grow in importance. Finally, consulting firms with specific expertise and knowledge are in high demand and are being recruited to help organizations meet the demands of a rapidly changing industry.

Rob Casalou has seen firsthand how the healthcare management career progression has evolved:

> When I was coming out of school, the jobs were in operations. They were so hospital-centric 20 years ago that the physician office piece was almost an afterthought. The route to the CEO office is still there, but it has changed by virtue of the fact that healthcare has changed. Where operations experience is often coveted as a means to getting to the CEO office, now they are requiring that you know how a medical group works, how an accountable care organization (ACO) works, and they want to see that you have had black belt, green belt, or yellow belt training and that you can do process improvement.

The experience requirements are changing and thus the path followed by current CEOs is not necessarily the same path that will prepare you for the management position you're ultimately seeking. Although process improvement is a popular choice because you gain experience streamlining procedures in many different areas, you run the risk of becoming pigeonholed and you really aren't developing experience running or managing anything. With physician practice management you're managing and supervising people and working closely with physicians, but you aren't in a hospital setting gaining key exposure to hospital operations. With consulting you'll have the experience of working in many different organizations, but essentially you go in, do your job, and then leave. You don't get any experience with changing the culture of the organization or dealing with management issues related to change.

> *Once you get into process improvement you are in operations, because you're learning what it's like day to day.*

While recent graduates and others are finding jobs in these areas, it's important to understand that working in these areas can lead to such a level of specialization that a person can become pigeonholed. This term as it's used in the business world today basically involves a person being given a very specific task or scope of responsibilities and, as a result, developing only a particular skill. So, rather than knowing a little bit about a lot of subjects, someone who's been pigeonholed knows a lot about one or two very specific subjects.

While a narrowly defined skillset may be useful and important to an organization, it can be detrimental to someone trying to climb the healthcare ladder. If you spend too much time in a narrowly defined role, people will soon not be able to see you as anyone other than a "process improvement person" or "someone who knows a lot about the ambulatory setting, but doesn't know hospital operations" or "a consultant who, after modifying a process, isn't able to manage the cultural side of change."

So how can you avoid becoming pigeonholed if you go into one of the three most chosen areas? Does it mean that you should avoid them all?

Of course not!

Process improvement, physician practice management, and consulting are the growing fields and will provide many jobs in the years to come. Also, becoming pigeonholed isn't exclusive to these three areas, so even if you work in another discipline you'll still need to be mindful of how long you've been performing a specific role and continually find ways to add new skills to your toolkit.

To understand how to leverage your experience in one of these three popular and growing areas, I asked the CEOs the following questions:

> If becoming a CEO is the end goal, which is the best area for an early careerist to start working in: process improvement, physician practice management, or consulting?

> What are the advantages and disadvantages of working in each area?

> Do you feel that people who go into these areas risk being pigeonholed and, if so, how can someone break out of that mold?

The CEOs agree that experience in these three areas will provide you with valuable skills and knowledge, and they strongly encourage you to proactively manage your career and leverage your experiences to help you continue to climb the ladder and avoid becoming pigeonholed.

Process Improvement

Due to narrowing margins, changes to healthcare payment structures, and a struggling economy following the 2008 recession, process improvement, or doing more with less, became a critical skill and competency for all healthcare organizations. While the names of process improvement tools have changed over the years, from Business Process Re-engineering (BPR) to Toyota Production System (TPS) to Total Quality Management (TQM), and now Lean and Six Sigma, the concepts remain the same. In general terms, the purpose of process improvement is to remove all nonvalue-added time or "waste" from a process and reduce variation in the outputs. These tools are valuable to an organization's bottom line and, therefore, gaining experience in implementing them will benefit you greatly as you move up the ladder.

David Callecod says that

> Process improvement is a good route to go because you're going to be able to learn about processes and departments throughout the entire healthcare system. You may be solving problems from Purchasing to OR flow and turnover. So I think it is a much better and broader-based training ground than maybe managing a physician practice.

Garry Faja adds that

> A good route for people coming out of school today is to get into Lean process improvement rather than a role like strategic planning. Once you get into process improvement you are in operations, because you're learning what it's like day to day. It's also a great way to get exposure to how things are done and how you can improve things, which really should be the role of a general administrator.

Although working to implement process improvements will allow you to gain great experience in a variety of different departments and disciplines, you're not managing people and you're not ultimately responsible for the success or bottom line performance of a department. As a result, early careerists are being advised as soon as possible to find a role managing people and a budget, which is considered operations experience versus solely working in process improvement. In an effort to heed this advice, many early careerists elect to go into physician practice management.

When I asked Jack Weiner about the advice to manage people and a budget as soon as possible, and if going into process improvement will get you pigeonholed and not allow you to own a process outcome, he said,

That is hogwash! So you're telling me that if I give you Respiratory Therapy and Security, and now you have people and a budget and you go and do that for 2 years, or I can put you in process improvement where in the first 6 months you have to analyze, break down, and help the Director of Pharmacy redesign pharmacy processes, how they link with nursing, and how they link with the retail public community. Also, you will go and work in Radiology and figure out how to reduce turnaround time in radiology reports, which makes the medical staff happy and reduces the cost of transcription, and, by the way, you will complete two other projects in two other departments all within the first year. Now if you were to sit down with the CEO and COO to interview for an entry-level VP of Operations role, who do you think they are going to hire? On the one hand, you had 40 people that reported to you, but were any of them nurses, pharmacists, or professional people?

Speaking to how long someone should stay in a process improvement role, Garry Faja suggested roughly 3 years:

> You need to make it clear that your objective is to gain as much exposure as you can to the ins and outs of day-to-day operations so that you can become a general administrator. This is how you avoid being typecast and let them know that you don't want to go into this job to become a process improvement person for the rest of your life. You are doing it to learn and so you need to be clear about this.

Jack Weiner says that he'll put someone into a process improvement role for about 2 years and then pull him or her out:

> If you go into an organization and they say that they want a 5-year commitment in process improvement, then run! Two to 3 years is a good timeframe, and then you should say that you would like to move into a new area and maybe do process improvement part time. Then, with the other half of your time, you should try to take on a couple of special projects like clinic development or leadership over a new service line that the hospital is looking at.

The point Jack is making is that after you have been in the role for a while, you should try to transition out and find new ways to enhance your value.

David Stark adds that

> I would not advise someone to stay in a process improvement role for longer than 2 years past their fellowship. That is the hurdle point of

saying that's kind of who you are. You're the process improvement guy and it's hard to say that you can then go run radiology or handle surgery, plant ops, and maintenance or run a service line.

While process improvement may be a good first step and expose you to a lot of different areas, the CEOs advise that, if you spend too much time in this type of role, people will begin to see you only in that light and you'll have to work hard to convince them that you can move into other areas.

An example of taking your career into your own hands and breaking out of a process improvement mold is Peter Karadjoff, who worked as a management engineer for about 4 to 5 years. Peter says people would tell him on a regular basis that he was doing a good job in his role, but after nearly 5 years he decided that he wanted to do something different:

> So I began interviewing outside the organization and was actually offered a job as the Director of Management Engineering at another organization. When I went back to my organization and announced that I was going to leave, they said, "Well, we told you that you were doing a good job!" Well, I know you told me that I was doing a good job, but you're not doing anything about it.

> "I would always try to get into a role where you're supervising people because you're going to have to learn process improvement anyway."

Peter felt that he needed to take his career into his own hands and make things happen. As a result, his current organization made a counter offer and Peter decided to stay with them, taking on a role in ambulatory services management. Once his organization knew that he was interested in doing more and that he was willing to leave in order to do so, they gave him opportunities in different areas and he was able to keep his career moving. Peter was so serious about leaving that he was even looking for houses in the new area. He cautions that if you're going to give notice that you're going to leave, then make sure you're serious and can follow through in case your organization doesn't decide to make a counter offer.

Physician Practice Management

Working in physician practice management allows you to develop valuable and practical experience managing people and working closely with physicians. Precisely for this reason, some of the CEOs, such as Quint Studer, recommend an early careerist begin to chart his or her path in physician practice management versus process improvement:

> I would always try to get into a role where you're supervising people because you're going to have to learn process improvement anyway. But if you just do process improvement, then you're going to be viewed as a specialist and could pigeonhole yourself. Practice management is a great place because you're showing that you can work with physicians, you can understand reimbursement and revenue trends, and you're going to have to be good at process improvement. I think process improvement is no different than being able to run a good meeting and no different than being able to read an expense report. Our problem in healthcare is not process improvement. We know what processes are better processes; it's implementing those processes.

Quint adds that too many young people go into positions that may get them a slightly better title and a little more money early in their career, but they will pay the price later on because they won't be able to take it to the next level:

> As a specialist you will be on a faster career track till you're about in your mid-30s, and so this is not a bad job if you don't want to become a CEO someday. But if you do want to be a CEO someday, or close to a CEO, it's all about how you lead people, not how you lead processes.

Quint shared an example of a young man who, after graduating from a master's program, went into management engineering. Early on in his career this young man met regularly with leaders in the C-suite and helped them with all types of management engineering issues. In the meantime, all of his buddies were in basic supervisor and manager roles. "Then one day, all of a sudden," Quint says, "he's 38 years old and his buddies are now vice presidents and he's the director of management engineering, because he never parlayed it. So I am a huge believer that you've got to show that you can lead people."

The point Quint is making is that when you're leading others you are naturally going to have to be good at process improvement to be successful. What is really important is how you lead your team to follow good processes and ensure that your team is doing the right things in the right way. Leading others is one of those skills where no matter how many management books you read, you'll never be truly good at it and understand just how hard it is until you're actually the person in charge. Leading others requires you to be consistent in your decision making and treat everyone fairly. It also requires you to engage in uncomfortable conversations when a team member is not performing up to expectations and to continually set an example for the rest of the team to follow. Your job is not to be the team members' best friend, but rather to lead and guide them toward achieving organizational goals and objectives. These skills are only developed and honed through real-life application and practice, and so developing these experiences early in your career will be critical to your success.

Similar to Quint, David Stark says that physician practice management provides a lot of value to early careerists, not just from the physician-exposure side, but also from the fact that you'll have an opportunity to really own something:

> Having accountability for a P&L statement and managing people and a budget is what you should be looking for. Demonstrating that you managed 25 people and a $1 million budget and hit budget every year means a great deal more in my mind than having helped operational improvement in the lab. This is good, but you probably didn't implement the improvement and you just moved on to the next project.

David adds that process improvement doesn't provide you with direct ownership of anything and that's what people are looking for in someone's career progression.

Physician practice management also gives you exposure to working with physicians in the ambulatory setting. Speaking to this, Gail Warden says,

> Taking a position as an office practice administrator for a few years will do two things for you. One, it will give you a really good picture of what goes on in the ambulatory care setting and will expose you to the delivery of primary and specialty care. Secondly, it will give you a really good feeling for working with physicians and what works and what doesn't.

Echoing Gail's comments, Peter Karadjoff says that practice management is a great way to understand how physicians function, and that this knowledge is critically important because physicians essentially feed hospitals. Peter had the opportunity to manage physician practices early in his career:

> I gained so much from those experiences that when I walk into a doctor's office, I can quickly look around and get a sense of how things are running. I also learned what their schedule is like and that being a doctor

isn't as glamorous as everybody thinks. You've got to realize that as a primary care physician you most likely graduated at the top of your high school class, at the top of your college class, you worked really hard in medical school, and competed to get into a residency. Then when you finally graduate, you go to the same building every day where you've got three exam rooms that you go between and you see about 30 to 35 patients a day. This can be very monotonous, and so I began to appreciate why a lot of doctors get burned out very quickly.

Graduate schools do not provide you with this type of real-world perspective and insight into a physician's life. Only through direct contact and working closely with them will you begin to truly understand their challenges and concerns. Additionally, physician practice management will allow you to take ownership of the outcomes of your decisions and to develop the leadership skills necessary to be a successful healthcare executive.

Consulting

Consulting is another great avenue to begin your career in healthcare management. In consulting you'll have the advantage of working in a lot of different organizations and settings, being exposed to an array of issues and challenges, and seeing how different organizations solve problems and address issues in a variety of ways. You'll learn many different ways of doing things and develop your own list of best practices.

Garry Faja, who worked as a consultant after graduate school, shares his experience:

> Working as a consultant gave me an opportunity to work in a lot of hospitals in many different settings. My work as a consultant was essentially process improvement, but it was process improvement in many different hospitals. So I got to see how everybody does things a little bit differently and how much the problems are the same. Additionally, I was exposed to different management styles and how things are done in many different hospitals. I got to see the small hospitals and I got to see the huge hospitals, and this was great exposure.

Kevin Unger also began consulting right out of graduate school and says it was the best experience he's had in his career:

> I was thrown into situations where I had to think on the fly and I learned skills about how to formulate strategies and put together my thought

process. Additionally, I got to sit at the board table with senior managers and see how they work and address issues. My projects were typically around 6 to 8 weeks long, and so the work was intense and I was always problem solving.

Kevin highly recommends going into consulting early in your career because you gain exposure to process improvement, strategic planning, and operations activities. Kevin also became familiar with many different aspects of healthcare by working with health insurance payers and hospital providers.

While the exposure to a variety of organizations through consulting is beneficial, it's important to understand that consultants only work in a particular setting for a short period of time and thus don't get experience managing the cultural effects of change. A potential employer may view this as a negative because change management is a critical skill that every executive must have. Individuals who choose consulting will need to be mindful of this and look for ways to develop experience managing change.

New graduates and early careerists who go into consulting will also be given roles to support the more senior partners, including information gathering, data analysis, and project management. Although these are great skillsets to have, you'll need to make sure that you can parlay them into a management and operations role in a hospital before too much time passes or, as with the other routes, you'll risk becoming pigeonholed.

> [I]t's not a question of where you start, but rather what you do next and how do you continue to build on that foundation.

Leverage Your Experiences and It Really Won't Matter

Process improvement, physician practice management, and consulting are all great paths to pursue and will provide you with incredible opportunities to learn and grow. It bears repeating, however, that you risk becoming pigeonholed if you focus on only one of these narrowly defined disciplines. For this reason, all of the CEOs recommend that you only stay in one of the areas for a few years and then move into another to continue your learning, development, and career progression.

So how do you choose which path is right for you?

The CEOs suggest that all three are good areas to start your career and ultimately you can be successful no matter which path you choose first, as long as you leverage your experiences and continually grow your skillset.

According to Nancy Schlichting:

> I don't think it matters where you start. You have to start somewhere and each of these will provide tremendous learning opportunities since working on process change is how operations are improved and working with physicians is a vital skill that you will need as well. So it's not a question of where you start, but rather what you do next and how do you continue to build on that foundation.

Nancy says that if you were to start in process improvement, then in a couple of years go and spend some time running a physician practice or clinic to get that experience as well. She explains that your career is like building blocks and so you need to figure out in what core areas you need to gain competency (process change, understanding physicians, leading others), and then look for opportunities to learn and build upon those skills.

Sean Williams says that having expertise in any of these areas will benefit you by providing you with a baseline skill that will allow you to get your foot in the door. He adds, however, that

> Within either of these areas, what you should be looking for in order to avoid being typecast is whether or not you are going to be able to lead and manage others. This is important because leading and managing is really irrespective of the particular discipline that you're in, and leading others is a process in and of itself that can be overlain on a hospital, a department, or a service line. So you always want to ask if there is a structure that will allow you to lead and manage others within that discipline.

Your ability to lead and manage others is what will ultimately allow you to successfully climb the healthcare ladder. For this reason it's critical that you continually look for ways to learn new skills, lead others, and leverage your experiences to avoid becoming pigeonholed.

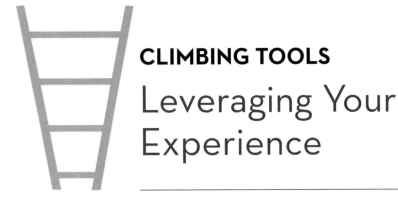

CLIMBING TOOLS

Leveraging Your Experience

- Whether you begin your career working in process improvement, physician practice management, or consulting, each will provide you with valuable experiences and skills. Proactively manage your career and leverage the experiences you develop in each area in order to transition into another area, expand your skillsets, prevent you from being pigeonholed in one area, and move your career forward.

- Working in process improvement you'll learn how to improve the operations of an organization as well as gain exposure to many different areas and departments throughout the entire healthcare system. You are not, however, developing experience managing people or a budget.

- Working in physician practice management will allow you to work closely with physicians and manage people, as well as expose you to the delivery of primary and specialty care. You are not, however, working in a hospital setting or gaining exposure to hospital operations.

Climbing the Healthcare Management Ladder: Career Advice from the Top on How to Succeed, by Jim Aldrich (Copyright © 2013, by Health Professors Press, Inc.)

- Working in consulting will allow you to work in many different organizations; be exposed to a variety of issues and challenges; and gain experience in process improvement, strategic planning, and operations activities. You are not, however, developing experience with changing the culture of an organization or dealing with management issues related to change.

- Work in process improvement, physician practice management, or consulting for a few years and then move into another area to continue your learning, development, and career progression.

- Remember that if you want to be a CEO someday, or close to a CEO, it's all about how you lead others, not how you lead processes.

Climbing the Healthcare Management Ladder: Career Advice from the Top on How to Succeed, by Jim Aldrich (Copyright © 2013, by Health Professors Press, Inc.)

SECTION 3

Enhancing Your Success

It's important to understand that the secret to turning a good career into a great career is to continually find ways to enhance your success. *Webster's* defines *enhance* as "to increase or improve in value, quality, desirability, or attractiveness." The key words here are *increase* and *improve*, which suggest that there is an existing foundation or knowledge base that you can add to or build upon.

This foundation or knowledge base is developed in school, where everyone essentially learns about and is exposed to the same issues and concepts. It is upon graduation when people begin to diverge in terms of level of knowledge and variety of experiences. This is when new graduates can decide whether they've learned enough and only want to focus on the skills needed to perform their current job or if they want to continually seek out new experiences to broaden and enrich their knowledge base.

The CEOs in this book fall into the second category. Throughout their careers they've looked for ways to gain new experiences, grow their skillsets, and expand their knowledge to enhance their success and accelerate their climb up the healthcare ladder.

This section discusses the actions that the CEOs took to enhance their success, including the following:

> Developing strong relationships with mentors and regularly
> seeking their advice

Learning how to work effectively and develop strong partnerships with physicians

Making a concerted effort to focus on professional development

Understanding what life is like as a CEO and maintaining a healthy work–life balance

These key actions allowed the CEOs to increase their value to their organization, improve the quality of their work, and enhance their desirability and attractiveness to future employers. By following the CEOs' advice in this section, you'll be able to turn a good career into a great career.

11

Mentors

Whether you're a student, early careerist, VP, CEO, or even retired, we all need mentors to help guide us throughout the various stages of our careers. Due to the circle of life, there will always be someone who has been in your shoes and dealt with the challenges, questions, and concerns you're facing in charting your career path. So it's critically important that you take advantage of their knowledge, learn from their mistakes, and ask for their advice. Not doing so could be the difference between leading a productive and successful career or one that is full of unfulfilled potential and avoidable mistakes.

Due to the critical role that mentorship will play in your career, it's important to understand that there are many types of mentor relationships. For example, in a formal mentoring relationship one person is assigned to be someone's mentor and they meet on a regularly scheduled basis. In contrast, and much more common, is informal mentoring, in which one person seeks advice from a more experienced person from time to time. The discussions are not regularly scheduled and the two parties involved probably don't even view themselves as a mentor or a mentee. Yet another form is indirect mentorship, by which you simply observe and learn from how others around you respond to and handle certain situations. If you observe someone handle a situation either poorly or in a positive manner, you'll know better how you would want to behave or react in a similar situation.

Throughout your career you will most likely engage in each of these types of mentor relationships and perhaps even all three at the same time.

Regardless of how successful you've been or how busy you are, everyone needs mentors from time to time and thus these types of relationships should be sought out and embraced. Speaking to this, David Stark says,

> Securing a mentor is critically important and will offer a consistent guide throughout anybody's career. No matter if you're a student or a seasoned 25-year CEO, everyone needs one at different stages. You may need different things from them, but you still need one.

To understand how the CEOs benefited from and continue to benefit from mentors, I asked the following questions:

What makes a mentor relationship successful?

Who should you look for to be a mentor and how do you choose the best mentor for you?

How did you benefit from your mentor relationships?

While no two mentor relationships are the same, there are very clear strategies and actions that you can employ to help make these relationships as effective and fruitful as possible, including finding people who will tell you the truth, carefully choosing the right mentors for you, and effectively managing these relationships to ensure that you're learning and growing from them.

Will Tell You the Truth

An important part of the mentor relationship is finding people who will be honest with you and tell you the truth about which areas you need improvement in to advance your career. Mentors such as this are beneficial, according to Jack Weiner, "because too many mentors tell you what they think you want to hear because they want to be nice. The person who will help you the most is the one who will tell you the truth, as much as you don't want to hear it." Jack went on to say that when people who ask him to be a mentor and don't ask him to be brutally honest in that role, they're telling him that they just want someone who they can put on their résumé as a reference who will say nice things about them. Jack says,

I'll do this, but I'm not going to spend a lot of time with them and I don't feel it's going to be very productive. The person that comes to me and says, "I want your job, tell me what I need to do or what I need to change in order to get that," is the person that I will bend over backward for.

Similar to Jack Weiner, Kevin Unger says that you want someone who's looking out for your best interest and will give you the straight scoop:

You want someone who is on your side but isn't going to blow smoke at you. They are going to tell you their opinion and give you the straight news, regardless of whether it's good or bad. These are the kinds of people you want to align yourself with and spend time talking to.

Gail Warden benefited throughout his career from the honest and truthful advice of his mentor, Walter McNerney:

Walter was very up front about things and always told me what he thought. When I had been at Presbyterian St. Luke's Medical Center in Chicago for 13 years, Walter said, "Gail, you need to get out of there, because you're never going to be the President. The President is always going to be an M.D., and so you need to move on and find something that's going to broaden your career."

Gail heeded Walter's advice to move on, and with his help was able to become the Executive VP of the American Hospital Association (AHA). After about 5 years of being in that role, Walter again told Gail that it was time to move on, saying "Gail, you've made your mark as the Executive VP of the AHA and now you need to go and be the CEO of your own organization."

This type of honest and straightforward mentorship from Walter McNerney benefited Gail's career tremendously by encouraging him to continually push himself to keep moving and learning new skills. Gail Warden succeeded in becoming the CEO of Group Health Cooperative and the CEO of Henry Ford Health System, and ultimately finished his career as a member of the Modern Healthcare Hall of Fame.

Choose Carefully

In addition to having mentors who will be honest and direct with you, it's important to make sure that you choose the best mentors for you. Rob Casalou says that when it comes to choosing a mentor you should look for an individual who you believe is on the rise and will be around for a while:

> You could pick someone who is older and they could be a great mentor, but they won't be there helping your career along 5 years from now. So part of your criteria is that you've got to make sure that you're attaching yourself to individuals that have some longevity and have the ability to pull you along with them as they progress.

Rob also notes that it's important to be mindful that the mentor relationship involves a two-way selection, and so you need to find someone who's going to want to invest the time and be willing to mentor you. Echoing Rob, David Callecod says, "The secret is to find someone inside your organization that is interested in mentoring, and in my experience it was pretty apparent who was willing to spend time with me and who I could learn from."

While finding someone who you think is going to be successful and is interested in mentoring you are key first steps, you also need to think about the direction you want your career to go and then ask yourself if you think that person will be able to provide you with the mentorship needed to help you get there. When I asked Carrie Owen Plietz who you should look for to be your mentor, she said,

> It depends on where the person wants to end up. In my situation, I knew that I wanted to be in hospital operations and wanted to move up toward senior-level positions. So I was really looking for a mentor who was in that position and who was very willing to be open about how they got to where they are.

"You shouldn't have just one mentor, and you've got to be willing to look at different mentors at different times."

This advice is important in that just picking a mentor because he or she has an important title does not mean the person will necessarily be able to give you the best advice. For example, if your goal is to be a hospital CEO, then asking a CEO of a health insurance company or a pharmaceutical company to be your mentor may not be very helpful. Yes, the person is a CEO and may be able to give you great advice, but he or she does not fully understand the ins and outs of hospital operations and the specific skillsets needed to be successful in that environment. Additionally, if your goal is to try and become a COO in the next 5 years, then you would be better served finding someone who is currently a COO to mentor you instead of asking a Chief Human Resource Officer or CFO. The mentor relationship will be more beneficial to your career progression if you find someone who has accomplished the types of goals you've set for yourself and whose experiences you can learn from to understand what led to his or her success.

While one mentor is good, more is better, and so you shouldn't limit yourself to just one at any given time. Speaking to this, Quint Studer says,

> You shouldn't have just one mentor, and you've got to be willing to look at different mentors at different times. Also, don't always believe everything you read or hear in the media, because sometimes in healthcare the leaders and organizations that get the most attention don't necessarily have the best outcomes; they just have the best publicists. So really try to look at the outcomes and make sure if you're going to pick a mentor that they truly are a good performer and get the right results, because you really want to learn from somebody who is having some success.

In addition to having multiple mentors who are having success, it's also important to learn from people at all levels, including your peers and direct reports. Denise Brooks-Williams has always had mentors at every level and enjoys being mentored by people who are where she wants to be, who are at her same level, and who she is leading. In a sense, Denise has engaged in 360-degree mentoring, in that the different perspectives really allow her to get a clear picture of herself and what she can improve on.

Speaking to how the mentor relationship works at different levels, Denise says,

> I have been fortunate to have had mentors that stressed development be formal in that we have good relationships and communication, but at the end of the day they force a real worldview of challenges. If you want to do "X," and there is a glaring gap, and how are you going to convince people that with that gap that you can still do the job and how do you sell your related experiences? When you're talking with your peers, you're trying to get a pulse of how they are doing and what they are going to do next and where they are seeing opportunities. Then for the people that I serve in a subordinate relationship, I ask them if I am serving them well, because your peers and mentors see you through one lens since they are not there working with you every day, but your

staff knows how things really are. So they are going to tell you like it is and they will tell you, "Hey, you're not giving me enough face time and you seem distracted." I want to hear these kinds of things because understanding how well I am serving them is going to help me improve where needed and prepare for the next level of leadership.

Similar to Denise, Peter Karadjoff feels that you can learn from everybody, and even the people who are your subordinates can teach you things. Speaking from the perspective of a CEO, Peter says,

Your CFO is going to be an expert in many things that you're not, and your CNO will be an expert in other things that you're not. So it's not always somebody up on a pedestal, and you're constantly absorbing from everybody around you.

The key point that Denise Brooks-Williams and Peter Karadjoff are making is that a mentor is not always a senior and more experienced person. In fact, *Webster's* defines *mentor* as a "wise and trusted counselor or teacher." There is no mention of age or seniority, and so it's important for you to continually learn from everyone around you and to be humble enough to admit when someone else knows more than you and then follow his or her counsel.

Inside or Outside the Organization?

Now that you know how to choose the best mentors for you, the next decision is whether they should be inside or outside your organization. While there is much debate on which is best, the general consensus among the CEOs is that having mentors both inside and outside the organization will provide you with the most value and broad range of perspectives.

> [H]aving that person on the outside to give you a true third-party perspective is valuable.

Having mentors within your organization is good because it's strategic and will help you gain perspective from leaders immersed in and familiar with your organization's culture. Additionally, mentors within your organization can potentially have some influence on your career by pulling you into new projects and providing you with new experiences. Speaking to the value of internal mentors, Kathleen Griffiths says,

If you have a supervisor or someone that you trust and respect and believe that you can learn from, then the more time you can spend with them asking for feedback and challenges, the better. Having a supervisor who will say, "I want you to go and do X," even though it might be pushing you out of your comfort zone, is really important.

While mentors inside your organization have their benefits, mentors on the outside can provide you with an unbiased third-party perspective and a safe environment to really open up and share your frustrations and concerns. Carrie Owen Plietz says,

It is good to seek mentorship outside the organization that you are working for because there are times when a situation will come up where you don't have a comfort level discussing it with somebody who may be at the same hospital or same organization as you. So having that person on the outside to give you a true third-party perspective is valuable.

It's important to choose mentors from both inside and outside your organization. This variety will provide you with an array of different perspectives and will allow you to have supporters inside your organization and confidants on the outside.

How to Make the Mentor Relationship Successful

Now that you have identified, chosen, and begun to seek advice from mentors, the easy part is over. You now need to continually manage and foster these relationships to ensure that you're learning and growing from them. Garry Faja suggests that one way to do this is to ask a mentor to watch you and give you feedback on how you handle a certain situation and to let you know how you could have done better. You should ask questions such as, "What could I have done differently in that meeting?" or "I didn't feel like that discussion went as well as it could have; what could I have done better?" Garry makes the point that mentorship doesn't have to take place in a formal office setting where the mentor is behind a desk while the mentee sits across from him or her asking question after question. Rather, mentorship can involve observation and asking someone you respect before a meeting to take notes on how you can improve your presentation style or group facilitation skills.

John MacLeod adds that you shouldn't be afraid to ask people to be your mentor. He suggests that you tell the person what your goals are and then ask, "Would you mind mentoring me for a while and may I ask you questions periodically or could we just sit and have a cup of coffee together once a week and talk shop?" John was approached like this by a young man who said, "John, I'd like to have your job some day and would you mind helping me get there?" John recalls, "I was proud of the fact that he asked me and so I have gone out of my way for the last 10 years to mentor him, and if things work out, some day he will be sitting in my chair." John says that he and his mentee still talk all the time. Since that initial discussion, his mentee has gone back to school to get his master's degree and is taking the steps necessary to achieve his goal of becoming a CEO.

Similar to how John's mentee approached him, Bob Milewski wasn't afraid to ask to be mentored. Bob had heard many great stories about Ken Meyers, who at the time was the CEO of Beaumont Hospital in Royal Oak, Michigan. He recalls,

> I am still surprised that I did this, but I went up and met his secretary and said that I would like to meet him. I was very young and naive, but I was able to meet him and he became a role model and mentor for me. It wasn't a heavy mentoring role, but over the years I have checked in with him many times, and whenever I had career choices to make I would go and see him and he would help advise and guide me.

In addition to asking for career-related advice, you should also use mentor relationships as sounding boards and opportunities to get counsel on issues you're currently facing and how your mentors would approach these situations. Speaking to this, David Stark says, "You should use a mentor to pick their brain about things, such as how do they handle certain situations, why do they approach things in the way they do, and what is their communication style."

Dr. Wayne Lerner adds that

> It is absolutely critical for you to find someone to be your sounding board as you progress in your career. This is not just for CEOs, but it is important for early and mid-careerists. You've got to have somebody who is going to speak to you clearly and definitively and say, "That just doesn't fly," "Don't rationalize it," and "Don't be passive aggressive."

Dr. Lerner says that all of these are normal reactions and that somebody has to be able to call you out on them: "It could be one of your good buddies, your spouse, your significant other, or a mentor. Regardless of who it is, you've got to have someone who will act as a sounding board for you and set you straight."

Informal Mentoring

While formal mentoring can be very effective in providing you with regular and consistent feedback, informal mentoring is by far much more common. This is probably due to the ease in which these relationships can be formed and dissolved. Also, with informal mentoring there are no strings attached, and a mentor and mentee can go months or even years without speaking to one another. Furthermore, these types of relationships have an open-door policy and allow the mentee to seek advice on an as-needed basis. While these relationships don't have the specific structure that a formal mentor relationship has, they nevertheless can be just as beneficial and valuable.

Nancy Schlichting says that sometimes people put too much emphasis on formal mentorship and not enough on informal mentoring. Early in her career she would watch people whom she admired to see how they handled various situations. Nancy never had a formal mentoring relationship, but she's had many great mentors over the years, some of whom even taught her things that she never wanted to do:

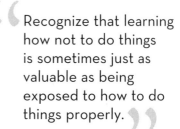

Recognize that learning how not to do things is sometimes just as valuable as being exposed to how to do things properly.

> There are mentors who are the negative people you deal with in your career that teach you those things that you want to avoid and the behaviors that you never want to emulate. They are important too, because you learn from all leaders—the good, the bad, and the ugly. Mentorship doesn't need to be structured and you just need to pay attention to those around you.

Similar to Nancy, Dave Spivey says,

> I think it's important to realize that you can learn and grow from both positive and negative situations and circumstances. So it is important that you take advantage of the learnings and practices you see being employed around you and begin to build your own philosophy and approach to management and leadership. It is important to recognize

that learning how not to do things is sometimes just as valuable as being exposed to how to do things properly.

While observing what not to do can be extremely valuable, it's more important that you find people you respect and make it a point to observe and learn from what they do. Speaking to this, Sean Williams says,

> Mentorship doesn't have to be a formal thing and you just need to find someone that you think is very good at what they do and then spend time watching what they do and how they act in certain situations. This is what I had the chance to do with my fellowship preceptor, Terry Penniman, and it was absolutely instrumental for me in terms of preparing me for everything from reading a financial statement to giving a board report to dealing with an upset family member.

Sean adds that you should look to someone who approaches the work–life balance the way you would want to approach it and who has the same ethical and moral framework as you. He feels this is important because as you observe someone over time, you don't realize until later just how much influence the person has had on you: "I still quote Terry all the time and I call them 'Pennimanisms,' because he had all these quotes that he used to use that would sum up different circumstances. I didn't realize until years later just how much impact those early influences would have."

Most informal relationships just happen naturally through the course of doing the work. Peter Karadjoff has had many informal mentors and each relationship started through projects he took on that allowed him to get to know each of his mentors: "The human dynamics of it are such that as you go through and do something and work on a project, you have a lot of human interaction and you're going to get to know people. It's hard to target someone and say I would like you to be my mentor. It's more informal and you get to know them through the course of doing the work." Peter adds that you shouldn't just pick people in positions of authority; rather, you should choose people you respect and think are smart and then try to pick their brain.

Pay It Forward

While mentorship is critically important to your career, it's also essential to the development and future success of the profession in general. The CEOs all said that they are grateful for their mentors and they try to return the favor by mentoring others. Speaking to this, David Callecod says,

> For the health of the profession, those who have had mentors need to be a mentor going forward. I have had almost 40 people now that have worked for me that I have mentored in some way and two of them are now CEOs of hospitals and numerous others are C-suite members in hospitals.

His mentoring relationships have been formal and some informal. Some have been part of graduate school hospital administration programs and others have been with people who have worked for him who wanted to move up and pursue administration. David says to those climbing the healthcare ladder,

> "Find yourself a mentor, and once you become successful, really seek out and be a mentor to others whenever you possibly can."

Jack Weiner has mentored 14 people who are running hospitals of their own. They have each given Jack a personal commitment to do the same for others. Jack says, "It's like having a family tree, and I want to be able to look back and say that I have 70 people who can be tied back to me who are running hospitals in the United States and are making a difference and are doing the right things for the people they're serving." Jack wants this to be the legacy and mark he leaves on healthcare.

So no matter if you're a student, early careerist, VP, CEO, or are retired, mentorship will play a critical role in your success. The CEOs strongly encourage you to take advantage of those who have gone before you by learning from their experiences and seeking their advice. Mentor relationships will be of great benefit to you and will provide you with the extra support and encouragement you need to successfully climb the healthcare ladder.

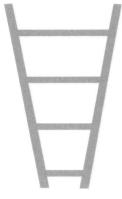

CLIMBING TOOLS
Mentors

- Find mentors who will be honest with you and tell you the areas in which you need improvement to advance your career.

- In choosing a mentor, think about the direction you want your career to go and find someone who will be able to provide you with the mentorship needed to help you get there.

- Don't limit yourself to only one mentor at a time; maintain a variety of mentors both inside and outside your organization in order to benefit from their unique perspectives and insights.

- Find mentors who you respect and admire and pay attention to what they do and how they handle various situations.

- Once you become successful, seek out others to mentor whenever you possibly can.

Climbing the Healthcare Management Ladder: Career Advice from the Top on How to Succeed, by Jim Aldrich (Copyright © 2013, by Health Professors Press, Inc.)

12

Working with Physicians

One of the single greatest factors that can impact the success of your career for either good or bad is how well you work with physicians. Effectively managing and fostering these relationships will allow you to gain their trust and be seen as a partner instead of an adversary. While no two physicians are the same and each has his or her own personal set of beliefs, values, and motivations, all physicians want to provide their patients with the best care possible. This is also the goal of hospital administrators. Why then is the physician/administrator relationship so often viewed as adversarial and negative? These two parties have the same goal and passion for helping patients, but due to unaligned processes and payment structures they're not pulling in the same direction and are often stuck trying to solve the same problems from very different perspectives. Adding to this struggle is the fact that most physicians do not work for the hospital and are paid based on the number of tests and procedures they perform. While physicians performing tests and procedures is certainly not a bad thing if they're what the patients need, healthcare costs are skyrocketing and thus need to be managed and controlled. The job of a healthcare administrator is to try and provide the highest quality of care at the lowest possible cost and in the most efficient manner, all while ensuring the highest levels of patient satisfaction.

So while physicians and administrators don't wake up each morning thinking about how they can make each other's lives difficult, the setup of the healthcare industry inherently puts these two parties in conflict. This doesn't have to be the case, however, as shown by the CEOs in this book who have been able to establish highly successful and productive working relationships with physicians.

I asked the following questions to understand how the CEOs effectively managed this critical relationship:

What has made you successful in working with physicians?

How do you establish relationships with members of your medical staff?

What are the key supports that physicians want from the hospital?

What Physicians Want

The key to successful relationships is knowing what others want and then giving it to them in the way they want. This is often the key distinction between the Golden Rule, which is to "Treat others how *you* would want to be treated," and what is known as the Platinum Rule, which is to "Treat others how *they* would want to be treated." This is a subtle difference, but it really speaks to the fact that all people are different and just because someone would want to be treated one way doesn't mean that someone else would want to be treated in that same manner. For this reason administrators need to view problems from the physicians' perspective and carefully consider what would be a successful solution to a particular issue.

It became very clear from my interviews with the CEOs that physicians basically want what almost everybody else does, including

to be treated with courtesy and respect,

to be able to come to work and perform their jobs without unnecessary delays and complications,

to be involved in the decisions that affect their daily work,

to be recognized and rewarded for doing a good job.

These may seem like very basic expectations, but if you keep them all in mind when working with physicians you'll succeed in developing strong working relationships with them and assist them in providing their patients with the best care possible.

Building Relationships Based on Courtesy and Respect

When asked how he develops relationships with physicians, David Stark said, "It's important to develop a personal relationship and have it not just be a 'hi' in the hall. I understood what they did, I knew sometimes what their family did, and I would take a personal interest in their lives." David would also spend time going out to their offices to understand what their clinics were like and what their challenges were. He committed to these efforts to have a better understanding of what he could do to help. David would also always leave by asking, "What else is there that I can help with?" and "Is there anything else I can try and figure out for you?"

Rob Casalou also makes it a point to develop relationships with physicians by visiting them in their office:

> Early on what I really try to do with doctors is to build a relationship first, because you'll never build that relationship around a bad issue. What you have to do is establish your relationships in a natural environment so that when the bad issue does come or something does come up, you've got that relationship to fall back on.

He says that you don't bring the doctors to you; rather, you go to them (to the floors, to the doctor's lounge, etc.). If a physician asks if he or she can come and see you, you suggest instead, "Let me come to your office, because my schedule is a lot more flexible than yours. I can catch you right after your office hours and then you won't have to walk all the way over." Rob says this may sound trivial, but it's the little things that speak volumes about how you're going to work with them.

Responsiveness and follow-through are absolutely critical.

Going to the physician's office not only shows that you respect the person, but also that you respect the person's time. Yet another way to be respectful of a person's time is to be up front and provide an answer right away, even if that answer is no. Speaking to this, Bob Milewski says,

Physicians are taught in medical school to be independent thinkers and decision makers in order to save lives. Sometimes they will have to make a snap decision, and especially that resident on the floor in the middle of the night when they are all alone. They have to make snap decisions and tough decisions that are life saving and critical. So they have zero tolerance for people who don't respond and move slow. The worst things you can do with a physician is to not answer a phone call or tell them you're going to have something by tomorrow and then not have it. So responsiveness and follow-through are absolutely critical.

The important point to understand is that physicians are trained to make quick decisions, whereas administrators are trained to try and build consensus and encourage buy-in from key stakeholders. As a result, administrators tend to overanalyze issues and can take a long time to make decisions as they deal with a lot of bureaucratic red tape. It's critical to be aware of this difference, provide physicians with as accurate a decision-making timeline as possible, and ensure that you follow through in a timely fashion.

Another way to develop strong relationships with physicians is to not only speak respectfully to them, but also to speak respectfully of them. Nancy Schlichting shares her experiences in this regard:

I have heard administrators in meetings complain about their physicians and it's like complaining about your children. If you're a kid, you know when your parents complain about you to their friends and it doesn't make you feel very good. The same is true when you're the administrator of a hospital and you're complaining about your docs all the time. Why do you expect them to gravitate to your organization if you behave like that?

Nancy makes the point that a culture of respect begins at the top with the hospital leadership team, and if they are complaining about physicians all the time, staff members will eventually hear and begin to openly complain as well. A culture of complaining quickly ensues and is readily apparent to members of the medical staff. The key point to understand is that, as with everyone else, physicians want to be respected in terms of what is said to them and what is said about them.

A final key aspect to understand in getting to know and respecting physicians is that they have a vested interest in the community and often will have been in the community for many years. It may even be the community in which they grew up. In contrast, healthcare executives tend to regularly move from job to job and from community to community in pursuit of new opportunities. It's essential that you respect physicians' ties to the community and involve them in improving the health of the broader community.

Speaking to this, Dave Spivey says,

> I think you have to remember that in healthcare we often think and are taught that we as healthcare administrators can see the big picture and have the capacity to think about the health of the broader community. You have to be very careful about this and about trying to portray yourself as some big-picture, community-oriented person. It can often come across as illegitimate to the medical staff, because they are the ones who have often grown up in the community and have been educated and set their roots down there. So it's important to remember that they were there before you got there, they are going to be there while you're there, and they are going to be there when you're gone.

Dave adds that some physicians are also small business people who are very dedicated to the health of their patients and the health of the community they serve. So it's important for you to acknowledge this and not overplay your "health system executive" perspective on what is best for the community.

Efficient and Effective Processes

While developing courteous and respectful relationships with physicians is important, unless the hospital is running efficiently and effectively, physicians won't want to practice there. For this reason, the administrative team must work closely with the medical staff to understand what processes are not working well and then be willing to do whatever it takes to fix them.

Quint Studer says that physicians want to work in an efficient hospital and know that processes are going to run the way they are supposed to because if the hospital is running behind, then the physician's schedule will be running behind as well. He adds that

> I find that most administrators think physicians are more difficult than they really are, when the reality is that we just frustrate the heck out of them. Being a doctor is like going to the airport 300 times a year and you get there at a certain time because the plane is supposed to take off, but when you get there, all too often, you're told that there will be delays. Also that other things will be running late and we are going to miss a whole bunch of other stuff too.

Quint is acknowledging the fact that a physician's time is very valuable because they make money based on the number of cases and procedures they perform. If a physician is stuck having to wait around for an operating room (OR) to be cleaned, then money is being lost (for the physician and the hospital). Additionally, the patient is getting upset having to wait, and any other procedures will end up having to be delayed as well. The physician may have to skip lunch to get back on schedule, only to have another hospital delay set the schedule back again. As a result, the physician may have to stay at the hospital until late in the evening and end up missing dinner with his or her family. So while a 15-minute delay in cleaning an OR may not seem like a big deal, if all of the ORs are consistently experiencing a 15-minute delay to be cleaned, then by the end of the day a physician's final procedure could start 2 hours later than was originally scheduled. While physicians certainly don't expect the hospital to be perfect all the time, they do expect delays and broken processes to be held to a minimum and will greatly appreciate any efforts you can employ to keep things running smoothly and efficiently.

An example of this is when Denise Brooks-Williams first began her role as CEO of the Battle Creek Health System. Denise said that her first strategy was to go out and meet with physicians, and so she started with those who were formal leaders in the organization and then with specialists who were highly dependent on hospital services: "I went to their offices as opposed to inconveniencing them to have to come to mine. I would also try to go with something, and so I would take them an update on the service or activity that was relevant to them, and then I would listen." Denise wanted to hear about what their experiences had been with the health system and to let them know that she was there to make things better or to keep processes the same if they were working well: "I didn't assume that they had had a good or bad experience. I wanted to hear what their experience had been, and if everything was going great then how do I keep that going, and if things could get better what could I do to help."

Denise understands the importance of providing physicians with an efficient and effective hospital to practice in, and so she regularly visits members of the medical staff to hear from them how processes are working and how she can make them better. By doing this Denise has gained the trust and confidence of her medical staff and shown them that she wants to be their partner in helping them to provide the best patient care possible.

When it comes to working with physicians, focus the discussion around patient care and how a certain process change will help to improve care. Speaking to this, Mike Slubowski says,

> First of all you have to get in their shoes and you have to understand that they have been trained as scientists. You've got to remember that at the end of the day, whatever biases you have about how much money they make, that fundamentally physicians are drawn to healthcare because they want to help people. It would be hard to believe that for some of them who are very financially oriented that they could live with doing that for 20 to 30 years unless at the end of the day they got some satisfaction out of taking care of people. So you always have to remind yourself that fundamentally there was a calling, and how do you acknowledge that calling in your work with them?

Mike adds that you need to keep the discussion focused on the patient and remember that healthcare is all about how physicians and healthcare organizations can come together as care partners for the patient's benefit.

Jack Weiner notes, "Graduate schools tend to create a 'we/they' mentality, and that your job is to fight with the docs and you've got to control and manipulate them to get them to do what you want." This is the worst outcome possible, because it should actually be about relationships and finding areas of mutual agreement and ways to work together. Jack adds,

> The best advice I ever got was if you can get the argument around how to improve patient care, that you'll never get an argument from a doc on trying to find a way to do that. If the argument is around how do I get the doc to do what I want, then it's going to be rare that you win. If you can place the question in terms of, "Doc, how can I help you do what's best for your patient?" then you'll never lose.

Involved in Decision Making

In addition to being treated with respect and having an efficient hospital to work in, physicians want to be involved in the decisions that affect their daily work. Nancy Schlichting has seen firsthand what happens when they are left out of a decision-making process:

> I see it so many times where administrators will bring physicians in at the last minute and then get ticked off when they don't jump on the

bandwagon for a particular project or change. You really need to get physicians involved early and make sure that their input has been sought and that you're listening. Additionally, the result you create should reflect those ideas or otherwise they are not going to feel like you really cared about their opinion.

When it comes to involving physicians in decision making, David Callecod has found that

> There are always one or two unofficial leaders of the medical staff that really kind of pull the strings of everybody else, and the secret to being successful is to try as quickly as possible to figure out who that person is. It is never readily apparent who has both medical and social influence over the other docs, but in every hospital there are one or two guys that behind the scenes are the influencers.

When I asked David how he approaches working with these one or two unofficial leaders, he referenced the expression "You should keep your friends close and your enemies even closer." David tries in general to spend a lot of time with them and makes sure they're involved in decision making.

While physicians say they want to be involved in decision making, they're all very busy and don't have time to pay close attention to every change the hospital is making. They're also usually on staff at several different hospitals and would never have time to attend all of the required meetings. For example, if a physician in Internal Medicine is on staff at three different hospitals and were to attend every possible meeting, he or she would have to attend 18 department of medicine staff meetings and 12 general medical staff meetings each year. That's 24 meetings a year (or 2–3 meetings each month), of which the majority are held outside normal business hours at either 7 a.m. or 6 p.m. In addition to these meetings, the physician would need to have the time to read the quarterly medical staff newsletters and the hundreds of other announcement flyers that litter the physician mailrooms and lounges. On top of all of this, some physicians are essentially a small business owner and so are constantly trying to make sure that their private practice is running effectively and efficiently.

So while physicians say they want to be included in the decisions that the hospital makes, in reality they do not have the time to weigh in on every one. Additionally, no matter how many times you communicate a potential change or how many ways you communicate it, there will always be people who say they never heard about it. The majority of physicians won't care what minor changes are taking place, just as long as it doesn't affect them or make their life more difficult. Whenever you're looking to make a change, try to engage in the process and seek the input of the small group of physicians who really drive the potential acceptance or rejection of proposals.

It's also important to regularly share the hospital's vision and strategic plan with physicians to ensure that they're on the same page as administration and know what the hospital will or will not invest in. According to Phil McCorkle, "As a CEO, you need to have a vision of where you

> " You really need to get physicians involved early and make sure that their input has been sought and that you're listening. "

want your organization to go, and the sooner you can interpret that and refine it so that the doctors know where you are going to take the organization, the better." If you leave physicians with too much doubt, then they'll start coming to you on a regular basis to request that the hospital begin offering some type of new service. It can then turn into a political nightmare if you say yes to one person and no to another. Phil offers the following response as an example of how to protect yourself from this type of situation:

> This is what we all agreed upon. We're going to focus on cancer and we're going to invest in neuroscience and orthopedics. These are our major centers of clinical focus. Additionally, we're working toward creating a large primary care network, and so everything we're doing has got to fit together. I can't start this program because it just doesn't fit with what we're doing and there are not enough resources. We can try to figure out how to include it within our strategic planning process and see if we can offer it in the future.

Phil adds: "It is vitally important to make sure everybody knows where you are taking the organization and that you are proactive and way ahead of them, or otherwise you set yourself up to be ambushed."

When involving physicians in the decision-making process, also ensure that they are getting a consistent message from all members of the leadership team. It doesn't matter if you're the CEO or not—if you're a part of the leadership team, it's your responsibility to communicate a consistent message to the medical staff or you'll cause confusion and frustration. Mike Slubowski says that there can be a tendency in some organizations for the physicians to always want to go to the CEO with any issues they may have. If a CEO is developing a good team and has given them the authority to handle various issues, then the CEO should not give different answers to physicians, thereby undermining the team's authority. Mike says that the CEO should try to mitigate issues by saying to the physician something along the lines of "I will look into this situation and I want you to know that I'm going to talk to Jim or Mary because I know that they are also very concerned about this, and then we'll get back to you together." Mike adds that, "If you let them do circles into your office and you overrule everything your team did that was right, then [the team members] start feeling disempowered." Mike has seen this happen in some organizations, where the COO or the administrator for professional services has said, "I know every time a doc doesn't like my 'no,' that they are going to run to the CEO, and he is just going to overrule it."

While this advice from Mike is directed to CEOs, it's critical that you understand that this does happen, and to succeed in working with physicians you'll need to make sure they're receiving a consistent message. You may have to be willing to have an open conversation with your CEO if he or she is undermining the rest of the administrative team, or you may even need to find another organization where you can be empowered to be successful. While this happens a lot at the higher levels, you should ensure that you're not undermining your own staff members. As long as physicians are receiving a consistent message, they can handle the answer "no." But as soon as the answer changes even once, you begin to create a lot of confusion and dissatisfaction.

Reward and Recognition

Physicians should also be rewarded and recognized for the great work they do. Speaking to the need for recognition, Quint Studer says, "People will often tell me that only about 1 percent to 2 percent of physicians on their medical staff are truly difficult, and then when I ask them what they are doing to reward and recognize the other 98 percent of the medical staff that aren't difficult, they say 'nothing.'" Unfortunately, the ones who get all of the attention from administration are the 10 or 12 physicians who are truly disruptive, never complete their medical records, throw things in the OR, and verbally abuse nurses. Hours and hours are spent discussing strategies for how their behavior can be changed and what the hospital can do to better serve them, when in all actuality the reason they act the way they do is because their behavior is tolerated and in the end they get what they want. While any administrator would say "this doesn't happen in my hospital," the fact is that it happens everywhere and it causes a great deal of dissatisfaction for those members of the medical staff who do follow the rules and behave as good citizens.

For this reason, just as managers are taught to give the most attention to their star employees, you will also need to give the most attention to the stars on your medical staff. It's human nature to want to be recognized for doing a good job, and any reward and recognition you can provide to physicians will go a long way.

There are many different formal and informal ways to reward and recognize physicians. It could involve creating a physician recognition board and hanging it in a high-traffic hallway with positive comments from patients. Members of the administrative team could send physicians handwritten notes to their home thanking them for the great work they do. Recognition could also come in the form of increased compensation or an appointment to a leadership role as a medical director or department chair. The list goes on and on, but the key is to find those physicians who are "good citizens" and who are contributing positively to the hospital, and then reward and recognize them in front of peers, family members, associates, the leadership team, and even the board. This will let them and the other members of the medical staff know that you appreciate their partnership and value their contributions.

> " I try to be positive about what it is that we are trying to accomplish and . . . recognize people for their contributions. I bring this same type of approach to our physicians. "

When Mike Slubowski was CEO of Providence Hospital, one example of an easy way he would recognize and develop relationships with physicians was by writing personal messages next to his signature when he had to send them their "renewal of privileges" letters. Mike recalls,

> There were a lot of these letters, and when I knew something personal about one of them, I would write a little handwritten note like, "Larry,

thanks for all you do for Providence and our ministry." I would write this off to the side of my signature on the letter, or if they were engaged in an initiative that I knew something about, I would put a note on the letter about that.

Mike says this was a very low-effort way for him to connect with physicians he might not otherwise see for a while. "It's just a minor thing," he says, "but it really makes an impact on somebody when you get a personal note, and it didn't take me all that much time to do."

Dave Spivey also understands the value of reward and recognition:

> People like to be recognized and to be acknowledged for their work and their contributions. Additionally, people like to be part of a team and to celebrate the successes of the organization and the initiatives that they work upon. So I try to be positive about what it is that we are trying to accomplish and very much recognize people for their contributions, and I bring this same type of approach to our physicians.

Physicians are extremely hard workers and make lifesaving decisions on a daily basis. The hospital could not function without them, and so it's important that you appreciate the work they do and reward and recognize those members of the medical staff who truly embody the mission, vision, and values of the organization.

As you climb higher and higher up the healthcare ladder, your relationships with physicians will become increasingly more important to your success. The decisions you make will carry more weight and thus will garner more attention from the medical staff. To ensure that the decisions you make and the relationships you establish are as effective and fruitful as possible, you will need to treat physicians with courtesy and respect, provide them with an efficient hospital to practice in, involve them in decision making, and regularly reward and recognize the great work they do. Doing these things will allow you to gain their trust, be seen as a partner, and enjoy a successful and prosperous career.

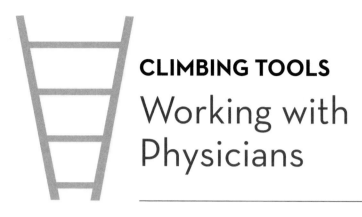

CLIMBING TOOLS

Working with Physicians

- Recognize that physicians want what almost everybody else does: to be treated with courtesy and respect, to come to work and perform their job without delays and complications, to be involved in the decisions that affect their daily work, and to be rewarded and recognized for doing a good job.

- Responsiveness and follow-through are absolutely critical in working with physicians, who are taught to be independent thinkers and decision makers in providing patient care and who, therefore, have zero tolerance for people who don't respond.

- Physicians want to practice in an efficient and effective hospital and so the administrative team needs to work closely with the medical staff to understand what processes are not working well and then be willing to do whatever it takes to fix them.

- It's essential that you respect physicians' ties to the community and involve them in improving the health of the broader community.

Climbing the Healthcare Management Ladder: Career Advice from the Top on How to Succeed, by Jim Aldrich (Copyright © 2013, by Health Professors Press, Inc.)

- When working with physicians, always focus the discussion around patient care and how a certain process change will help to improve care.

- Involving physicians early in a decision making process, making sure they are aware of the hospital's strategic plans, and providing them with a consistent message are critical to gaining physician buy-in.

- Be sure to reward and recognize the "good citizens" on the medical staff, instead of focusing all your time and attention on the disruptive 1 or 2 percent.

Climbing the Healthcare Management Ladder: Career Advice from the Top on How to Succeed, by Jim Aldrich (Copyright © 2013, by Health Professors Press, Inc.)

13

Professional Development

Due to the ever-changing nature of the industry, being a lifelong learner is a required part of the job for a healthcare leader. While it would be nice if everything you learned in school could carry you throughout your career, such is not the case, and so you'll need to continually look for ways to learn new skills and stay apprised of changes in the industry. Reading management books and journals, participating in professional organizations, and networking with other professionals will be critical to your development and will provide you with the tools needed to be successful.

It's easy to get overwhelmed with the required daily tasks of your job, and then when you also factor in family obligations, social commitments, and other commitments you may have in the community at large, your personal growth and development can quickly take a back seat to all of the other demands on your time. While your commitments to your family and current job are rightfully at the top, you also need to be sure to schedule some time in your calendar for professional development. This could mean waking up 30 minutes earlier in the morning to read an article from the latest healthcare journal or skipping your favorite weekend activity to attend a conference or seminar. As with anything, you only get out what you put in, and so when it comes to professional development, don't be stingy. It's an investment in yourself that has a high rate of return.

To understand how the CEOs managed their own professional development throughout their careers, I asked the following questions:

What books, journals, and other materials do you read to continually help you learn and grow?

How has your involvement in professional organizations aided you in your career?

How has networking helped you in your career?

The CEOs in this book recognized the importance of regularly focusing on their professional development and growth by reading numerous management books and journals, being active in professional organizations, and networking with colleagues throughout the industry. This focus allowed them to continually learn and grow throughout their careers.

Read, Read, Read

Thousands of books have been written about management and healthcare topics and hundreds more are written every year. With such a vast library to choose from, it's easy to get overwhelmed trying to decide which book to devote your precious free time to reading. To try and narrow the list down to a manageable choice of recommended reading, I asked each CEO to name two or three books that they considered a must read for all healthcare leaders. While there were a couple of books mentioned repeatedly, such as *Good to Great*, by Jim Collins, and *Hardwiring Excellence*, by Quint Studer, the CEOs recommended a very broad spectrum of books, ranging from the Bible to Sun Su's *The Art of War*.

> Whatever you read or watch, you can view it from a perspective of what does it teach me about management?

I quickly began to realize that it's not about trying to find the best management book ever written and then memorizing its pages. Rather, it's about reading a wide variety of books and then using what you learned to inform and develop your own management philosophy.

Speaking to this point, Dan Jones says, "There are a lot of books out there and what reading does is it allows you to bring perspective and it allows you to develop themes. One of the things that I would suggest is you should read across the spectrum instead of focusing in on one area." Dan compares this to politics, in that if you only read from the political spectrum that you affiliate with, then you'll never get to understand the perspectives of those on the other side. "So any time you read management books or any type of industry books," he says, "you always want to make sure that you get a good healthy perspective. Perspective is like a sphere, 360 degrees on three axes, and so you're trying to evaluate the situation from every vantage point."

Along similar lines, Garry Faja recommends that early in your career

> You should read as many management books as are available. The key is by reading those books you begin to create your own management philosophy, because many of these books are coming at the same thing with a little different angle. Some of them have good pearls of wisdom that you will want to keep and put into your own personal management portfolio. But what you've got to stay away from is being all about one book, because there are other books that are going to come forward over the years and different books float to the top. So if you like *Good to Great* and you say, well, the key thing about [the book] is the Hedgehog Concept, and then if you read *The 7 Habits of Highly Successful People* and say, well, five of those seven habits are really good and I like those. Now you're building your own portfolio of management.

In building your own philosophy, it's also important to look outside management books and see what you can learn from other fields or situations. One example of this is Dr. Wayne Lerner, who, when he was teaching a graduate management and organizational behavior class, would take a modern fiction work and ask the students, "What do we learn from this situation that teaches us about management?" Wayne explains that

> Whatever you read or watch, you can view it from a perspective of what does it teach me about management? Also, people need to start thinking about management not just from the silo of healthcare, but what can I learn from whatever I am reading or experiencing?

Like Wayne, Nancy Schlichting tries to read books outside healthcare and enjoys books about leadership:

> Throughout my career, I try to learn not just from healthcare but from nonhealthcare. I read *Fortune* magazine and all kinds of leadership books

that help me think about great leaders. When I was young I read about Henry Ford, Thomas Edison, Clara Barton, Helen Keller, and other people who had courage, because to be an effective leader you have to be able to take risks and you have to have courage. This comes from within, but you can aspire to it and you can learn from other leaders.

In addition to trying to create your own management philosophy, books provide you with an opportunity to strengthen your weaknesses. It's important to take a step back and ask yourself what your areas of weakness are or what opportunities for improvement do you have? Speaking to this, Carrie Owen Plietz says,

> You need to look internally and really conduct a critical analysis of what you believe or what other people believe are your strengths and weaknesses. Then read everything you possibly can to give you greater insight into strengthening those weaknesses.

Since there is no one-size-fits-all book out there, you'll need to read a wide variety and pick out the themes and concepts that resonate the most with you. As you do this, you'll begin to develop your own philosophy on management and, in a sense, write your own book on leadership.

Professional Organizations

In addition to reading books and journals, participating in professional organizations will allow you to learn new information, meet new people, and contribute to your professional development. Participation in these organizations is similar to putting money in the stock market. You only have a limited amount of money available to you and there are certainly many other ways you could spend your money that would bring you immediate pleasure and satisfaction. Furthermore, the stock market requires you to exercise faith that your sacrifice and investment will one day be worth more. Not every stock you invest in will make money, and so some stocks will be of more value to you than others. The hard part about the stock market is that you have to be patient in order to see any long-term changes, and you never know which stock will be the one that allows you to make it big.

The same is true with respect to participating in professional organizations. It takes a lot of faith on your part to add additional activities to your already full and hectic schedule. Not only are you giving up your free time to attend these events, but you also have to pay money out of your own pocket to attend. Furthermore, not every meeting, conference, or networking event you attend will teach you something new or introduce you to that next great contact. So some of these events will be worth your time and others will not. The challenging part is that you never know which event will be the one that makes a big impact on you and, just like the stock market, you often won't see results overnight. The key is that regular attendance and partici-pation in professional organizations over time will allow you to learn new information, meet new people, and, over the long haul, receive a return on your investment.

Get Involved

If you're not currently a member of a professional organization, then step one is to find out what's out there and join some of them. If you are a member of a professional organization, then get involved and don't simply pay the annual dues and fail to take advantage of the opportunities offered to you.

Speaking to the benefits of professional organizations, Denise Brooks-Williams says,

> They are a good way to get leadership opportunities, find mentors, and build upon your professional network. Many people say that their relationships with their professional organizations have led to job oppor-tunities, and so it's about keeping your networking connection very vibrant. There is not a one-size-fits-all organization and some people may not have needed a professional organization to be successful, but I think that it is important to use the formal structures that exist to help you continue to grow in the profession.

Carrie Owen Plietz strongly recommends that once you jump into a professional organization, don't jump out:

> You're going to get really busy, you're going to have a very full career, and you're going to have a personal life. But don't underestimate the benefit of networking, because the people who don't network find out just how much they need to network when something happens and they lose a job or the company transitions. So stay involved and have a strong network.

Carrie adds that a good way to get involved in a professional organiza-tion is to contact the president and ask how you can get involved and where they need help the most. She says that these organizations are always looking for volunteers, and if they can't come up with something for you to do, then that doesn't mean you can't jump in and make a recommendation. For example, you could offer to lead the early careerists committee and try and take that concept to the next level.

Peter Karadjoff had an opportunity to start a local chapter of the American College of Healthcare Executives (ACHE) in southeastern Michigan called the Midwest Healthcare Executives Group and Associates (MHEGA). He interviewed four to five chapters across the country to learn about best practices, and when he shared them with the local regent, he was asked to be the president of MHEGA. Peter recalls, "I had a family and a full-time job, but I did it and it was tremendously rewarding, and I remain very active in it today." He says that his membership in the local organization allows him to maintain his relationships and contacts. MHEGA brings in a variety of speakers, and since the meetings are local, Peter does not have to travel very far for an evening or breakfast meeting. This is important to Peter because he only misses an hour or two at the beginning or end of the day; he doesn't have to be out of the office for a day or two as he would if he were to attend a national conference. Being active and engaged in professional organizations has helped Peter form relationships and continue to develop professionally.

> " [It]'s about keeping your networking connection very vibrant. "

Variety Is Key

While any participation in professional organizations is beneficial to your career, participating in a wide variety of different organizations is what will really allow you to gain new knowledge as well as a broader perspective. Speaking to this, Betty Noyes says,

> Belonging to professional associations is very valuable for everyone, and I recommend that you belong to a lot of different types of associations. For example, I am a member of the American College of Healthcare Executives (ACHE), the American Society for Healthcare Engineering (ASHE), a human resource group, a Chief Learning Officer group, and an information systems group. This variety is so important. I recently went to an HR conference and I sat there and listened to the questions and the points of view of that particular segment of the market and it

was invaluable. Additionally, I get their newsletters and begin to pick up the nuances, and this is a very essential part of being credible.

In an effort to participate in a variety of associations, Betty tries to rotate which conferences she'll attend each year (e.g., she attends the ACHE Congress every 3 years or so).

Don Wegmiller also recommends that, in addition to joining the professional organizations in your field, you try to join other types of organizations that can bring you new perspectives:

> One way to do this is to get involved with local business groups. Early in my career I was a member of the Junior Chamber of Commerce (Jaycees). Later I joined the business roundtable in the Twin Cities, and so it's about getting out beyond your field and joining organizations that you think can really bring you information.

When it comes to professional development, we are all faced with the same time challenges in maintaining a work–life balance. Between your day job, family obligations, and other personal commitments, there is not much time left for professional development. Your professional development is, however, a continual must. The CEOs in this book all recognized the importance of professional development and invested their time and energy in reading management books and journals, participating in professional organizations, and networking with others in the industry. Just as in the stock market, they invested in the long haul and thus were able to enjoy a high rate of return and career success. Your challenge will be to do the same.

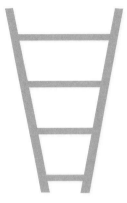

CLIMBING TOOLS
Professional Development

- Due to the ever-changing nature of the healthcare industry, being a lifelong learner is essential in becoming a healthcare leader.

- It's not about trying to find the best management book ever written and then memorizing it. Rather, it's about reading a wide variety of books and then using what you've learned to inform and develop your own management philosophy.

- Take a step back and determine what your weaknesses are or what opportunities for improvement you may have, and then read everything you can to give you greater insight into strengthening those weaknesses.

- Participation in professional organizations is a good way to develop leadership opportunities, find mentors, and build upon your professional network.

- Participating in a wide variety of organizations will allow you to gain new knowledge as well as a broader perspective.

Climbing the Healthcare Management Ladder: Career Advice from the Top on How to Succeed, by Jim Aldrich (Copyright © 2013, by Health Professors Press, Inc.)

14

Life as a CEO

Many people climbing the healthcare management ladder often feel stressed, overworked, and burned out. While this is true for most industries, a career in healthcare is one with many unique challenges. Workers are faced daily with life and death situations, razor thin margins, and continually changing rules and regulations. While those at each step of the healthcare ladder experience these challenges, they increase exponentially as you get closer and closer to the top. Like a thick fog covering a mountain peak, the healthcare ladder is ringed by competing demands for limited resources, endless challenges, and an unrelenting pursuit of perfection.

Those farther down the ladder typically don't see this fog. They may instead see the CEO coming or going, giving a speech for a groundbreaking, or meeting important people. They may also hear about how much the CEO is getting paid or even be envious of all the perks and advantages he or she seems to enjoy. What they don't see are all of the personal and family sacrifices that the CEO makes and the daily struggle for a work–life balance. They don't see the emergency phone calls and last-minute meetings that take place during what should be a relaxing family vacation. They don't see how the CEO feels on the inside when he or she shuts the office door to be alone and weigh the pros and cons of an unpopular decision. And they don't see the mental wear and tear the CEO constantly feels from the weight of thousands of other people's lives on his or her shoulders.

This chapter focuses on the life of a CEO, because having an understanding of this lifestyle will benefit your career greatly. Having a glimpse into this life will allow you to self-reflect and decide if this type of position is truly something that you want to work toward. Having an understanding of the struggles and challenges faced by CEOs will also allow you to understand where they're coming from and how you should approach various issues and challenges.

To learn more about what life is like as a CEO, I asked the following questions:

What are the pros and cons of being a hospital CEO?

How do you maintain a work–life balance?

If you could go back, would you do it again?

Whether or not your goal is to become a CEO some day, having an understanding of the CEOs' daily struggles and challenges will allow you to put yourself in their shoes and add value to the things they care about.

Time Commitment

A CEO's time is in constant demand from board members, physicians, staff members, patients, families, the corporate office, and members of the community. As a result, he or she is constantly being pulled in many different directions and is required to work long hours, wear many different hats, and continually move from one topic to the next.

When I asked Kevin Unger what an average week is for him in terms of number of hours and evening meetings, he said,

> I average 70 hours a week and I am out probably 3 nights during the week. Every day is started early and rarely after 7 a.m. Night meetings involve meeting with physicians, community members, and attending other events. The docs like to meet early and late, and I'm also regularly giving talks and updates about the hospital to the community.

Alan Channing says,

> Being a CEO is a very challenging and demanding experience. I typically work 7 days a week, not 8 to 12 hours 7 days a week, but every day I

am working. This involves being in the community, doing paperwork at home that I never have time to get done during the week, and coming in on weekends and in the evenings to make rounds in the organization in order to sustain that visibility. It also involves participating in community activities so that the community sees me as the committed face of the organization.

Rob Casalou faces the same demands on his time: "An average day is 10 to 12 hours, and so it's a 60-hour week. Now, throw in some dinner meetings once or twice a week and it's probably closer to 70 hours a week." Rob adds that you also have weekend commitments, social functions, golf outings, holiday balls, and lots of other ceremonial activities that will regularly require your time and participation.

> " Being a CEO involves long hours, lots of stress, and being pulled in different directions. "

From the CEOs' comments, it's clear that this job will require long hours and a lot of personal sacrifice. This is the nature of the job, and no matter how good you are at managing the work–life balance, being a CEO comes at a cost and you'll have to determine if you're willing to pay that price. Speaking to this, Jack Weiner says,

> Being a CEO involves long hours, lots of stress, and being pulled in different directions. You've got your normal work life, you've got the community that's expecting you to be an active participant, and you've got the political environment. You've got good compensation and you'll live better than most, but most importantly you get a chance to go to work every day and do something different and make a difference. If the ability to do that is worth the price you pay, then it's a great job. If the ability to do that is not that valuable and it's about the money, then go into finance, because you'll make more money and you won't have those pulls on your life."

Jack adds that there are tradeoffs; you may have to miss some baseball games and you may not be there for every concert or school activity, because you're at the hospital until 11 p.m. opening a new unit or attending a medical executive committee meeting that went late. "People need to understand that there are tradeoffs," he says, "and if you think it's an 8-to-4:30 job and then you just go home and live your normal life, forget about it. You can't do it, and 60-hour work weeks are relatively standard."

Also speaking to the demands on your family life, Mike Slubwoski says,

> You don't have much of a personal life, so you and your family have to have a conversation about how you're going to balance family responsibilities and make them work. The reality is, as a COO, or CEO, your meetings with the doctors are going to start early, at 6:30 in the morning, and you're going to have meetings at 6:30 at night. So your days are going to be long, and you can't turn it off because you're going to get called or you're going to be on call, and there is always going to be some crisis or some meeting that you're preparing for.

Mike also notes that there are many events you'll need to attend that will consume a lot of time. So you need to plan on at least a 70-hour week, and you've got to have those upfront conversations with your family regarding the demands on your time during the week.

While a standard workweek for a CEO is about 60 to 70 hours, mentally it's more like a 168-hour workweek. A CEO's job is never done and so you'll need to be accessible 24 hours a day, 7 days a week. Speaking to this, Dr. Wayne Lerner says,

> If you want to be a CEO of a hospital, it is 24/7 and you have to be willing to assume that responsibility and know that you never are off. Even when I am on vacation, I am never far away from work. You have to be willing to accept that responsibility and understand that the organization is your responsibility all of the time.

Commenting on the immense feeling of responsibility, Bob Milewski says that the higher up the ladder you get, the more demanding the job becomes, especially the step from COO to CEO, where the job suddenly becomes your whole life:

> All the responsibility rolls up to you and you can never turn it off. You just feel so responsible, and every time I would drive in or out of the parking lot I would look and see all those cars in the lot and I would think about all the lives and all the patients, babies, and families that come to this hospital for care.

Bob was CEO of Mount Clemens Regional Medical Center in Mount Clemens, Michigan, which at the time was a 300-bed hospital with about 2,500 employees. At times, he would consider how many lives the hospital was touching, that it was probably close to hundreds of thousands, if not a million lives each year in one way or another. Bob adds,

In addition to patients, it's family members, friends, co-workers, their dependents, and others coming to your hospital, and so you're touching a lot of people's lives, and that is a huge responsibility and you just can't shut that off. You're kidding yourself if you think that you're going to become a CEO and it's going to be an easy job.

Noticeably Absent

In addition to the tremendous feeling of responsibility, the CEO is also the face of the organization and is expected to regularly participate in community events. For example, Phil McCorkle, who is the CEO of Saint Mary's Health Care in Grand Rapids, Michigan, says that if he feels tired one night and decides to skip a community event, rather than saying "Phil didn't come," the community will say "Saint Mary's Healthcare

> " You want to make sure that you're a part of the fabric of the community. "

didn't come, and I guess that organization doesn't care about this particular cause or initiative." A CEO's time is not his or her own; he or she must always be promoting and representing the hospital. Phil says that attending community events is also about maintaining relationships in support of programs, initiatives, and fundraising:

> For example, Grand Rapids, Michigan, is one of the most philanthropic cities in the United States. So there is always some type of fundraiser or recognition dinner going on almost every week, and it's all about supporting relationships.

Many prominent people give millions of dollars to the hospital to help support new programs and initiatives, and so Phil feels that he ought to be there when someone is being recognized as "person of the year" or "philanthropist of the year" or for an event someone may be hosting. He says, "You want to make sure that you're a part of the fabric of the community, and so participating in those kinds of events is really important."

Work–Life Balance

With constant demands on their time and with only 24 hours in a day, it's no wonder that CEOs struggle to maintain a healthy work–life balance. According to Kevin Unger

It's a very demanding job and always will be if you're going to do it well. So trying to figure out where to draw the line between your personal life and your professional life I think is a struggle for pretty much everybody that I talk to. You've just got to carve out time and prioritize and make sure family is really the reason that you're here.

Life as a CEO and maintaining a healthy work–life balance can be made easier by having a great administrative assistant, scheduling time with your family, and remembering that it's a team effort of you and your spouse or partner.

Administrative Assistant Is Key

Don Wegmiller says that being a CEO will take more time away from your family and other interesting pursuits, more so than for anybody else in the organization:

> This is not good, but it is the nature of the job. There are lots of constituencies that expect you to spend time with them and that's understandable, but it comes at somebody else's time and that's usually your family and your friends.

When asked how best to balance work and family, Don recommends that you budget your time, take specific time with your family, and always plan for vacations. Having a highly skilled and efficient assistant is the most effective means by which Don can achieve a work–life balance:

> It's important to have an executive assistant who understands that you need to have time other than work time. So they are not just efficient at scheduling your work time, but are equally as efficient at preventing your family or personal time from being encroached upon. Some assistants are better than others and some love to give away your time, because they are rewarded, thanked, and appreciated for it, and then you're the one that suffers.

Don adds that the assistant you want is the one who will say, "There's going to be a good cop and a bad cop here, and I'll be the bad cop. People won't love me and they maybe won't appreciate me, but I'm going to do the job that you ask of me and I'm going to protect your time."

Bob Milewski says that in addition to having an administrative assistant who protects and controls your calendar, you need someone who doesn't make you feel guilty in trying to satisfy everybody else's demands for your time:

> It is absolutely essential to have somebody who protects you and looks out for you. Additionally, you need someone who is able to tell people no, but knows the stuff that you have to be at, because there are some things that you just politically and career-wise can't miss. So it's important to have someone who can sort out the difference and protect your time and schedule.

Schedule Your Balance

Scheduling your balance means setting aside specific time for you to spend with family and to do other activities. Speaking to this, John MacLeod says that

> There is no such thing as an 8-hour day for a CEO, and if I work an 8-hour day, I would consider that a short day. You just have to balance that workload, and so on Thursday afternoons I try very hard to be out of the office by 3:30 p.m. to play golf at my country club.

John doesn't always make it, but he has his administrative assistant block his calendar on Thursdays at 3:30 p.m., and the only ways that he doesn't make it are for corporate meetings or emergency meetings with a physician or someone else. So for John golf is a relief, and he says that you have to specifically schedule these types of activities to have balance in your personal and professional life.

Understanding the importance of a work–life balance, some CEOs go so far as to put fake meetings on their calendar so they can make sure they are home with their family on a Friday night or are able to attend a child's school play. Some of the CEOs said that even their administrative assistants don't know that these meetings are fake and their calendar will say something like "Dinner with Dr. Jones," when in reality they're going home to spend time with their family. The CEOs agree that a sustainable work–life balance does not happen unless you schedule it.

> " A sustainable work–life balance does not happen unless you schedule it. "

Another strategy is to look for untraditional ways to spend time with family. Denise Brooks-Williams says that often as a CEO she will have to leave for work before her kids wake up and return home after they have gone to bed. To find a balance, Denise says, "I try to make a time for my kids and it may be untraditional time, but sometimes it might be that I go to the school in the middle of the day and surprise my girls at lunch, because I didn't see them go to school and I know that I am not going to see them when I come home." Denise adds that you just need to find any way you can to keep all of your priorities in order.

Tom Priselac recommends that you first reconcile yourself

> to always having a nagging sense that you don't have balance. But I have found that people can and do truly make the time to do those things they really find important. So during the last 16 years that I have been a CEO, and as a COO for 10 years before that, while my two sons were growing up, I always made it a point to coach their soccer team and their little league baseball team and the other kinds of things to make sure we had as much interaction and balance in that regard as possible.

Rob Casalou says that you need to promise yourself that you're not going to miss baseball games and other events your kids may have:

> Even if I am talking to a doctor who is angry with me and says that he has to see me right away, I will say, "Well, doc, I have to see you tomorrow night, because it's my son's baseball game tonight," and there is no one who wants to tread on that.

Rob adds that the 30 year old who is working tons of hours and is trying to grow to become "CEO of the world" is making a big mistake in not spending time with family, because 20 years from now he or she is going to be 50 and look back and ask, "Was that all worth it, and was it worth missing my kids grow up?"

It's a Team Effort

Yet another strategy for achieving a work–life balance is to include your spouse or partner in as many events as possible. When I asked Phil McCorkle how he manages being out two to three evenings a week, he said, "You better have a spouse that doesn't mind going along." A CEO and his or her spouse or partner need to work as a team.

Rob Casalou strongly advises that your spouse needs to become a part of your job:

My wife is deeply integrated into my job and she is now chairing the holiday ball and she is at the hospital quite often. You and your spouse have to do it as a team, and this is what will keep your marriage strong.

Challenges

If the time commitment and work–life balance issues haven't scared you from wanting to be a hospital CEO yet, there are many other challenges that are unique to the position. Speaking to this, Don Wegmiller says,

> The buck always stops with you, and if there is a patient incident in your hospital, then you're accountable. Whether you were there or not, it's your accountability, and if the nurses in your organization decide to go on strike, it's your responsibility to see that patients get care. You do have people helping you, but if it doesn't work out, you're the accountable person, and this can be very wearing.

Echoing Don, Dr. Wayne Lerner says that you need to recognize that the institution is yours, the bad or the good:

> Your job is never done, and when you walk the halls of the hospital and there are messes on the floor, you've got to pick them up because all of the messes are yours. In the end, the bad stuff is yours while the good stuff is due to the work of your staff.

For this reason, Wayne says that you've got to be comfortable with putting the spotlight on others and not on yourself:

> I am constantly amused how some CEOs think it's all about them. I don't think anybody comes to my hospital because I am the president. They come to my hospital because of my doctors, my nurses, the other professionals, and the woman at the front desk. That's why they come to my hospital. The CEO needs to be able to put him or herself in the right frame of reference. We are simply blocking guards whose job is to open up a hole in the line so people can run through it and do their job!

The CEO must accept that something could go wrong at any minute and when it does, everyone is going to look to him or her for answers. So while everyone can have a friendly relationship with the CEO and help contribute to the organization's success, at the end of the day all of the responsibility falls on the CEO's shoulders. Speaking to this, Dan Jones says,

> Being a hospital CEO is a very lonely role and there is nothing more affecting than the first time the door shuts and you're in your office and you have to make an important decision and there's nobody to turn to but yourself.

He recalls that the biggest surprise when he became a CEO was just how lonely the role is. The role is classically visible and highly involved, but it's lonely in the sense that there's not that camaraderie anymore and there's a distance that occurs between you and your team. Dan adds that it's incumbent upon the CEO to make sure that he or she cultivates and feeds those relationships and keeps them strong, while also ensuring that there's a level of authority and a clear delineation of decision making.

And when it comes to making the tough decisions, Mike Slubowski describes it as having

> the weight of the world on your shoulders. You have a responsibility for thousands of people and they are depending on you to lead and make the right decisions. Additionally, when you make decisions about downsizing, you're affecting people and it just tore at my guts every time we had to go through those kinds of changes and knowing the impact. It really moves you after you have been through that.

All Eyes on You

Another challenging aspect of being a CEO is one that most people don't think about or aren't even aware of. It is the constant feeling of always having to be "on" and that everyone in the organization is watching your every move. The truth is, everyone *is* watching the CEO. Everything from how the CEO treats others in meetings to whether he or she picks up garbage off the floor and even how he or she dresses informs the rest of the associates about what is permitted and what the culture is going to be. For this reason the CEO and other senior leaders need to understand that every little thing they do is under a microscope and that they are constantly being watched by associates, board members, physicians, and even members of the community.

Speaking to this, David Stark says,

> The higher up you go in the organization, the more people watch you and everything you do. Where you eat dinner, where you park, what you wear, and how you interact with people. They take a lot of cues, whether you realize it or not, and they watch how you interact in a meeting, do you pay attention to folks, and they watch your activities very closely. You live in a glass house the higher up you go in the organization and it takes some getting used to.

Peter Karadjoff says that the job is bigger than you and that you need to be mindful of the power of the position. Especially in a small town, being the CEO of the hospital draws attention. Peter cautions, "It's important to remember that it's not you but rather the role that has the element of celebrity. So you're always on."

Positives

Now that I've painted a picture of doom and gloom, why would any rational and sane person want the job of CEO? When asked why anyone would want to be a CEO, Dr. Wayne Lerner said,

> Because you are able to move an organization and help it succeed and evolve. You are able to contribute to the community, have a positive impact on people's lives, and provide a venue for jobs in communities where jobs are not plentiful. You are able to watch people grow and progress and mentor people to move into broader leadership roles. You are able to see the kinds of changes that quality efforts have and see the effects of all these actions. There can't be any greater joy in life.

Nancy Schlichting says that everybody wants to have meaning in life, and she can't think of a more meaningful role than to lead a hospital organization or health system:

> We touch human life in all aspects from the beginning of life to the end of life. We try to constantly improve the care and support we provide to people who are dealing with incredibly difficult life situations. Additionally we work with amazingly talented and diverse groups of people and it's like running a small city. You learn every day, you contribute every day, and it's never boring. It's just fantastic and I still love it every day.

Alan Channing adds that

> Every day you have an opportunity to impact other people's lives and improve the health status of a community. Additionally, the kinds of things that a hospital executive gets to do in a week's time or even a day's time can cross the spectrum from worrying about how to keep the floors clean to worrying about the latest medical technology. There are few other jobs that I've seen that have that kind of array of activity.

Mike Slubowski appreciates how multifactorial and fascinating the job is. He hasn't had a day where he's woken up and not been excited about going to work:

> There are a variety of things that you do as the leader. I can have a day where I am focusing on how are we going to prioritize a $100 million capital budget to a patient complaint phone call that makes it all real. So the thing that makes it all worth it is the variety of what you're engaged in, the number of connections and relationships you are developing, and the bounce between strategy and operational reality, and how you keep all of these things in check while also framing everything around a bigger picture and direction. It's inspiring to see the progress of people in their development and to see success for the organization in improving its quality or financial performance. You just get a big kick out of seeing that movement that doesn't come overnight, and it's very inspiring and gives you the energy to keep going.

Similar to Mike, Dave Spivey says,

> It's tremendous to be able to be the leader of an organization and have the capacity to create a cultural environment. Additionally, to be able to move an organization forward and see it grow and develop and improve in its objectives to serve the health needs of a community is very rewarding and more than makes up for the work that you have to put in to achieve it.

As you have no doubt realized by now, the job of a CEO is never done and requires a significant level of commitment and personal sacrifice from those who take up this mantle of responsibility. One of my favorite quotes that speaks to this is from American essayist and naturalist John Burroughs: "For anything worth having one must pay the price, and the price is always work, patience, love, and self-sacrifice."

The CEOs in this book worked incredibly hard to achieve their success, and having obtained the top job they continue to work harder than ever before to serve the organization, their associates, and the community at large. So while the CEO role may appear glamorous to you now as you begin to climb the healthcare management ladder, upon closer inspection you'll quickly discover competing demands for limited resources, endless challenges, and an unrelenting pursuit of perfection. At the top of the ladder you'll also find incredibly dedicated, devoted, and passionate individuals who, despite all of the challenges they face, would do it all over again.

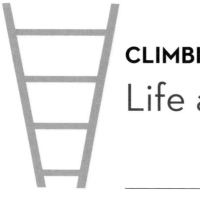

CLIMBING TOOLS
Life as a CEO

- As a CEO, you'll constantly be pulled in many different directions and be required to wear many different hats. The job of CEO requires long hours and a lot of personal sacrifice in managing the work-life balance.

- To maintain a work-life balance as a CEO, you'll need to be intentional about scheduling time to spend with your family or participate in other activities.

- Your job as a CEO is never done—the organization is your responsibility at all times. Anything that goes wrong in the organization is your responsibility and anything that goes right is because of your associates.

- As a CEO, everyone will be watching you, and everything you do will inform the rest of the organization about what is permitted and what the culture is going to be.

- Your life as a CEO will be fascinating and will allow you to have a positive impact on thousands of people's lives and improve the health status of a community.

Climbing the Healthcare Management Ladder: Career Advice from the Top on How to Succeed, by Jim Aldrich (Copyright © 2013, by Health Professors Press, Inc.)

NOTES

1. American College of Healthcare Executives. Retrieved January 6, 2011, at http://ache.org.

2. Richard G. Scott. (October 2010.) The Transforming Power of Faith and Character. Available at http://www.lds.org/general-conference/2010/10/the-transforming-power-of-faith-and-character.

3. MindTools.com. The Conscious Competence Ladder: Making Learning a Happier Experience. MindTools.com. Available at http://www.mindtools.com/pages/article/new ISS_96.htm. Reproduced with permission.

4. Carl Bialik. A Lifetime of Career Changes. The Numbers Guy, *Wall Street Journal* blog. Posted September 3, 2010, at http://blogs.wsj.com/numbersguy/a-lifetime-of-career-changes-988/.

5. James M. Citrin and Richard A. Smith. (2003.) *The Five Patterns of Extraordinary Careers: The Guide for Achieving Success and Satisfaction.* New York: Thunder's Mouth, pp. 109, 111.

6. Jacob Morgan. Working Hard vs. Working Smart and the Myth That Young People Are Told. Posted December 28, 2010, at http://www.jmorganmarketing.com/working-hard-working-smart/#.

7. Jon Gordon. The Benefits of Hard Work. Posted November 9, 2009, at http://www.jongordon.com/blog/2009/11/09/the-benefits-of-hard-work/.

8. Mike Dixon. Do You Spend 80% of Your Time Communicating? Posted February 10, 2011, at http://www.cmoe.com/blog/do-you-spend-80-of-your-time-communicating.htm.

9. Stefan Anitei. 10 Amazing Facts about Human Speech. Posted February 7, 2011, at http://news.softpedia.com/news/10-Amazing-Facts-About-Human-Speech-70397.shtml.

10. John Maxwell. Today's Word Is *Relationships*. Posted March 25, 2011, at http://johnmaxwellteam.com/relationships/.

11. Peter F. Drucker & Masatoshi Ito Graduate School of Managment. About Peter F. Drucker. Claremont Graduate University Web site. Available at http://www.cgu.edu/pages/292.asp.

12. Gary Martin. To Be, or Not to Be, That Is the Question. The Phrase Finder Web site. Available at http://www.phrases.org.uk/meanings/385300.html.

13. American Hospital Association. Fast Facts on U.S. Hospitals. Available at http://www.aha.org/research/rc/stat-studies/fast-facts.shtml.

Contributor
Gallery

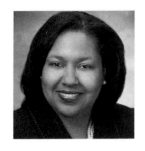

DENISE BROOKS-WILLIAMS
President and CEO, Henry Ford Wyandotte Hospital

CEO EXPERIENCE

2/2013–Present	Henry Ford Wyandotte Hospital	Wyandotte, MI
7/2011–1/2013	Bronson Battle Creek	Battle Creek, MI
9/2009–6/2011	Battle Creek Health System	Battle Creek, MI

EDUCATION

Master of Health Services Administration
University of Michigan, Ann Arbor, MI

B.A. Psychology
University of Michigan, Ann Arbor, MI

BACKGROUND

Brooks-Williams is president and CEO of Bronson Battle Creek, a 218-bed inpatient acute care hospital. She joined Battle Creek Health System in 2009 as its president and CEO. She has 20 years of senior executive healthcare leadership.

She began her career as a management fellow at Mercy Hospital in Detroit. She worked at Detroit Medical Center and Mercy Hospital, strengthening the operating performance in numerous areas, including physician networks, ambulatory development, and advocacy. She also served as Vice President of Operations for Ancillary and Diagnostic Services and Oncology Program Development at St. Joseph Mercy Oakland in Pontiac.

She has been active in numerous professional groups, including serving as president of the National Association of Health Services Executives (NAHSE), a premier minority health professional organization. She serves on the boards of several organizations and is engaged in the promotion of growth and diversity in the healthcare profession, including serving as a board member of the Institute of Diversity and serving as the alternate delegate to Regional Policy Board 5 of the American Hospital Association's Section for Health Care Systems.

Among her honors, she received NAHSE's Young Health Care Executive of the Year Award and the Early Careerist Award from the Michigan chapter of the American College of Healthcare Executives (ACHE). In 2010, *Modern Healthcare* magazine named her one of the Top 25 Minority Executives in Health Care.

Brooks-Williams lives in Battle Creek, Michigan, with her husband and two daughters.

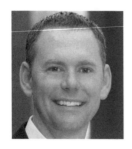

DAVID L. CALLECOD
President and CEO, Lafayette General
Medical Center

CEO EXPERIENCE

7/2008–Present	Lafayette General Medical Center	Lafayette, LA
11/2003–7/2008	Marion General Hospital	Marion, IN
12/2001–11/2003	Central Arkansas Hospital	Searcy, AR
7/1998–7/2001	Winona Memorial Hospital	Indianapolis, IN

EDUCATION

Master of Business Administration
Indiana Wesleyan University, Marion, IN

B.S. Communications Wabash College
Crawfordsville, IN

BACKGROUND

Callecod became President and CEO of Lafayette General Medical Center in July 2008. Under his leadership, LGMC has experienced rapid improvement in patient satisfaction and quality measurement, all while expanding the hospital itself, its regional network, and its award-winning care.

Since 2009, LGMC has received numerous awards, five-star ratings, and national rankings for orthopedic surgery, prostatectomy, overall gastrointestinal services, general surgery, and patient safety. Inpatient satisfaction at LGMC has steadily climbed, reaching the 99th percentile in June 2011. In 2011, he was inducted into Studer Group's Fire Starter Hall of Fame for his ability to keep the true spirit of an organization alive and flourishing, while achieving phenomenal results in short spans of time.

While he was President and CEO at Marion General Hospital, the hospital saw record patient satisfaction and quality measures as well as Top 100 Hospital Awards in 2007 and 2008. MGH also received several HealthGrades Five-Star awards during his tenure and Magnet Hospital Status in 2008.

He began his career in 1989 at AMI Culver Union Hospital and then served as CEO at Tenet Healthcare hospitals in Indianapolis, IN, and Searcy, AR.

He is a Fellow of the American College of Healthcare Executives (FACHE) and received their 2005 Regent's Award as an outstanding healthcare executive.

Callecod and his wife are the proud parents of a daughter and two sons.

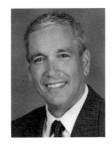

ROBERT F. CASALOU

President and CEO, St. Joseph Mercy Hospitals–
Ann Arbor, Saline

CEO EXPERIENCE

10/2008–Present	St. Joseph Mercy Hospital–Ann Arbor	Ann Arbor, MI
10/2008–Present	St. Joseph Mercy Hospital–Saline	Saline, MI
10/2008–Present	St. Joseph Mercy Hospital–Livingston	Howell, MI
7/2006–9/2008	Providence Park Hospital	Novi, MI
2/2000–6/2006	Providence Hospital	Southfield, MI

EDUCATION

Master of Health Services Administration
University of Michigan, Ann Arbor, MI

Master of Business Administration
University of Michigan, Ann Arbor, MI

B.S. Economics
University of Michigan, Ann Arbor, MI

BACKGROUND

Casalou joined Saint Joseph Mercy Health System (SJMHS) in October 2008 as the President and CEO of St. Joseph Mercy Hospitals–Ann Arbor, Saline, Livingston. Prior to coming to SJMHS, he served as President of Providence Park Hospital and was responsible for overseeing the construction of the 200-bed, full-service teaching hospital in Novi, MI, that opened in September 2008.

He sits on the Michigan Health and Hospital Association Board (MHA), served as chair of the MHA Legislative Policy Panel, and is a former member of the MHA Task Force on Hospital–Physician Alignment. He is a member of the American Heart Association (AHA) board, the AHA Advocacy Committee, and the AHA Child Obesity Committee. He also serves on the boards of Huron Valley Ambulance, IHA, Saint Joseph Regional Medical Center, the Center for Digestive Care, and Midwest Healthcare Executives Group and Associates (MHEGA) Board of Directors. He served as Chair of the MI CON Commission Standards Advisory Committee (SAC), the Greater Detroit Area Health Council (GDAHC), the Washtenaw Countywide Planning Steering Committee, the University Musical Society Corporate Council, and the Ann Arbor/Ypsilanti Chamber Board.

He is a member of the American College of Healthcare Executives.

Casalou and his wife reside in Novi, MI, with their three children.

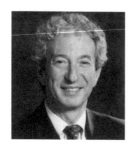

ALAN H. CHANNING
President and CEO, Sinai Health System

CEO EXPERIENCE

9/2004–Present	Sinai Health System	Chicago, IL
9/2003–9/2004	Channing Consulting Group	New York, NY
3/1998–9/2003	St. Vincent Charity Hospital	Cleveland, OH
7/1991–12/1997	New York Downtown Hospital	New York, NY
6/1989–6/1991	Bellevue Hospital Center	New York, NY
10/1986–6/1989	Elmhurst Hospital Center	New York, NY
1/1985–9/1986	Wishard Memorial Hospital	Indianapolis, IN

EDUCATION

Master of Health Services Administration
The Ohio State University, Columbus, OH

B.S. Business Administration
University of Cincinnati, Cincinnati, OH

BACKGROUND

Channing, FACHE, is President and CEO of the Sinai Health System, a three-hospital integrated delivery system on the west side of Chicago serving diverse inner-city communities that focuses on community health improvement. He has led financial turnarounds in three urban hospitals while improving their quality, expanding their medical staffs, enhancing their philanthropic activities, and recruiting new board members.

He is an assistant professor for The Ohio State University graduate program in healthcare management and has co-authored two books, *A Career Guide for the Health Services Manager* and *Really Trying*. He has published several articles on healthcare management, including The First 90 Days of Your New Job (*Healthcare Executive Magazine*, [2000]). He has presented testimony to federal and state legislators regarding hospitals and access to care. He has served as faculty for the JCAHO and has received the Senior Executive Award from the ACHE. He has served on the Regents Advisory Committee for northeastern Ohio and metropolitan New York.

Channing currently serves as the chairman of the Illinois Hospital Association and the chair of the board of a Medicaid Managed Care company. He is a frequent speaker on community-oriented health interventions and addressing disparities.

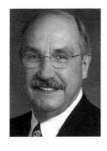

GARRY C. FAJA

President and CEO, Saint Joseph Mercy
Health System, Southeastern Michigan Region

CEO EXPERIENCE

1/1997–Present	Saint Joseph Mercy Health System	Ann Arbor, MI
1/1991–1/1997	St. Joseph Mercy Hospital-Ann Arbor	Ann Arbor, MI

EDUCATION

Master of Hospital Administration
University of Michigan, Ann Arbor, MI

B.S. Industrial Engineering
University of Michigan, Ann Arbor, MI

BACKGROUND

Faja is the President and CEO of Saint Joseph Mercy Health System, a six hospital system in Southeastern Michigan that includes St. Mary Mercy Livonia, St. Joseph Mercy Livingston, St. Joseph Mercy Ann Arbor, Chelsea Community Hospital–Chelsea, St. Joseph Mercy Oakland, St. Joseph Mercy Port Huron, and associated programs, services, and health centers. He has been affiliated with the system since 1982.

He has served as a delegate to Region 5 for the American Hospital Association and Past Chair of the Michigan Health and Hospital Association (MHA).

Faja is active on numerous Trinity Health and MHA committees and has served on numerous community boards.

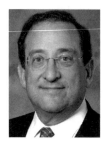

DAVID FINE

President and CEO, St. Luke's Episcopal Health
System

CEO EXPERIENCE

6/2004–Present	St. Luke's Episcopal Health System	Houston, TX
9/1999–6/2004	University of Alabama at Birmingham (UAB) Health System	Birmingham, AL
10/1990–7/1999	Tulane University Medical Center	New Orleans, LA
1/1987–1/1990	University of Cincinnati Hospital	Cincinnati, OH
1/1983–1/1987	West Virginia University Hospitals	Morgantown, WV

EDUCATION

Master of Hospital Administration
University of Minnesota School of Public Health, Minneapolis, MN

B.A., Economics
Tufts University

BACKGROUND

David Fine serves as President and CEO of St. Luke's Episcopal Health System. He has 38 years of experience as a healthcare executive, including more than 25 years as CEO of university hospitals, multi-hospital systems, medical groups, and managed care organizations.

Prior to joining St. Luke's in June 2004, he was CEO of the University of Alabama at Birmingham (UAB) Health System. During his tenure, UAB managed publicly and privately owned healthcare delivery assets, comprising $2 billion in net patient revenues, 11,000 employees, and 800 physicians.

He is past Chairman of the Board of the Association of University Programs in Health Administration, was founding Vice-chairman of the National Center for Healthcare Leadership, and is a past Regent of the American College of Healthcare Executives (ACHE). He is currently a Director of the Accreditation Council for Graduate Medical Education and Past Chair of the Commission on Accreditation of Healthcare Management Education.

Fine received the Birmingham Business Journal Health Care Executive of the Year in 2003, the Robert S. Hudgens Medal of the American College of Healthcare Executives, of which he is a Fellow, the Martin Luther King Special Humanitarian Award of the University of Cincinnati, and the Champion of Public Health Award of Tulane University.

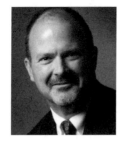

JAMES G. FITZPATRICK

Senior Vice President, Network Management and
Develop, Mercy Medical Center-Des Moines

CEO EXPERIENCE

5/2002–3/2012	Mercy Medical Center–North Iowa	Mason City, IA
12/2001–5/2002	Mercy Medical Center–North Iowa (interim)	Mason City, IA
6/1990–10/1999	Kossuth Regional Health Center	Algona, IA
4/1988–6/1/1990	Eldora Regional Medical Center	Eldora, IA

EDUCATION

Master of Health Services Administration
University of Iowa, Iowa City, IA

B.S. Public Affairs
University of Arizona, Tucson, AZ

BACKGROUND

FitzPatrick is currently the Senior Vice President of Network Management and Development for Mercy Medical Center–Des Moines. Since 2001, he has served as President and CEO of Mercy Medical Center–North Iowa. Prior to that, he served Mercy–North Iowa as the Senior Vice President of Network Development for 2 years.

During his tenure, FitzPatrick's accomplishments have been numerous and have created long-lasting, positive effects that will benefit the organization for years to come. Under his leadership, Mercy–North Iowa

- was among the first hospitals in Iowa to implement an electronic health record system (Genesis, 2005);

- was named a Top 100 Hospital for 8 years based on overall organization performance, including patient care, operational efficiency, and financial stability;

- was an advocacy force that impacted state and federal legislation that benefited the direction of healthcare and the lives of patients;

- established a new emergency department as well as a cancer center.

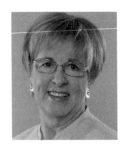

KATHLEEN GRIFFITHS
Retired

CEO EXPERIENCE
1/1998–1/2012   Chelsea Community Hospital   Chelsea, MI

EDUCATION
Master of Public Administration
New York University, New York, NY

Master of Social Work
University of Michigan, Ann Arbor, MI

B.A. Liberal Arts
Siena Heights College, Adrian, MI

BACKGROUND
Griffiths is retired as President and CEO of Chelsea Community Hospital in Chelsea, MI. She was with the hospital for over 30 years, serving as COO prior to her appointment as CEO in 1998.

She is a Fellow of the American College of Health Care Executives and has served on numerous nonprofit boards, including the Michigan Hospital Association, Huron Valley Ambulance Company, Chelsea Wellness Foundation, Arbor Hospice, Red Cross, and others. She continues on the board of Chelsea State Bank.

Since her retirement in January of 2012, Griffiths has been engaged in numerous volunteer activities and is a consultant for Washtenaw Community College serving as liaison between the college's healthcare programs and area healthcare providers.

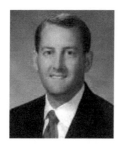

DAN JONES

CEO EXPERIENCE

9/2009–11/2010	Ochsner Health System	New Orleans, LA
5/2008–9/2008	Phoenix Baptist Hospital	Phoenix, AZ
9/2008–8/2009	Quorum Health Resources	Charlotte, NC
2/2004–12/2007	Centerpoint Regional Medical Center	Independence, MO

EDUCATION

Master of Health Services Administration
Virginia Commonwealth University, Richmond, VA

B.S. Economics
Randolph-Macon College. Ashland, VA

BACKGROUND

Dan Jones is an accomplished healthcare executive with more than 17 years of demonstrated success working in large hospitals, multi-campus health systems, and physician practice management roles. He has extensive experience in operational and clinical improvement, strategic development, and medical staff and physician relations, working with national and regional organizations such as HCA, Quorum Health Resources, Tenet, and Ochsner Health System. Various hospital medical staffs have recognized him for his support of and dedication to improving care and enhancing medical staff and employee relations.

He is the recipient of the American College of Healthcare Executives' Robert S. Hudgens Young Healthcare Executive of the Year award in 2006. The award was established as a tribute to ACHE's first vice president (elected office), by the alumni association of the Department of Health Administration at Virginia Commonwealth University. It is awarded to recognize young professionals for outstanding achievements in the field of healthcare management.

Dan Jones participates and leads in many community activities and organizations, including the Boy Scouts of America. He is an avid reader, enjoys spending time with his family, and is an accomplished private pilot.

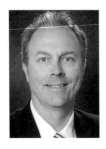

PETER J. KARADJOFF
President, Providence Park Hospital

CEO EXPERIENCE

5/2012–Present	Providence Park Hospital	Novi, MI
8/2003–4/2012	St. Joseph Mercy Hospital–Port Huron	Port Huron, MI

EDUCATION

Master of Business Administration
Wayne State University

B.S. Manufacturing Administration
Western Michigan University, Kalamazoo, MI

BACKGROUND

Karadjoff has 26 years of experience in healthcare and was appointed President of Providence Park Hospital in Novi, MI, in May 2012. An important part of his role is to continue to grow and expand services for the hospital and the surrounding communities that it serves.

He has a long track record of hospital leadership in the southeast Michigan market, and spent his entire career in Catholic healthcare, including 12 years in leadership positions at Providence Hospital in Southfield. Prior to his current position, he served as President and CEO of St. Joseph Mercy in Port Huron.

He is the American College of Healthcare Executives (ACHE) Regent for Michigan, and past President of the Midwest Healthcare Executives Group and Associates (MHEGA). He is also an ACHE Fellow.

Karadjoff is married and has two children.

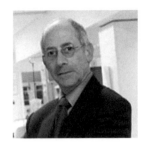

WAYNE M. LERNER
President and CEO, Holy Cross Hospital

CEO EXPERIENCE
4/2007–Present	Holy Cross Hospital	Chicago, IL
10/2006–4/2007	Holy Cross Hospital (interim)	Chicago, IL
4/1997–8/2006	Rehabilitation Institute of Chicago	Chicago, IL
9/1990–3/1996	Jewish Hospital of St. Louis	St. Louis, MO

EDUCATION
Doctor of Public Health Policy
University of Michigan, Ann Arbor, MI

Master of Hospital Administration
University of Michigan, Ann Arbor, MI

B.S.
University of Illinois, Champaign, IL

BACKGROUND
Dr. Lerner, DPH, FACHE, has more than 30 years of experience in healthcare administration, public policy, and education. He currently serves as President and CEO of Holy Cross Hospital, a 331-bed faith-based hospital serving more than 450,000 residents on the southwest side of Chicago. His efforts focus on stabilizing the hospital's precarious financial situation while addressing the health disparities extant in its primary service area.

He was a member of the U.S. Department of Veterans Affairs' Special Medical Advisory Group (SMAG), and is a Fellow in the American College of Healthcare Executives (ACHE), and the Institute of Medicine of Chicago (IOMC). He is past Chairman of the Board of the Illinois Hospital Association (IHA), as well as past Chairman of the American Hospital Association's (AHA) Committee of Commissioners.

In 2007, he received the Illinois Hospital Association's Excellence in Service. The University of Michigan's Department of Health Management and Policy honored him in 1995 with the *Lawrence A. Hill Award for Excellence in Health Management and Policy*. In 1986, he was elected one of the *AHA Health Care Leaders for the 21st Century*.

Dr. Lerner and his wife have five children and three grandchildren.

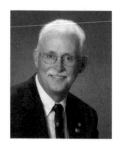

JOHN L. MACLEOD

President and CEO, Mercy Hospital

CEO EXPERIENCE

7/1999–Present	Mercy Hospital	Cadillac, MI
2/1992–7/1999	Otsego Memorial Hospital	Gaylord, MI
1/1978–1/1985	Clare Community Hospital	Clare, MI

EDUCATION

Master of Healthcare Administration
University of Minnesota, Minneapolis, MN

B.S. Business Administration
Central Michigan University. Mount Pleasant, MI

BACKGROUND

A former Lieutenant in the U.S. Navy, MacLeod has more than 35 years of experience in hospital administration. He has served as the CEO of Mercy Hospital in Cadillac, MI, since July 1999. Under his leadership, Mercy Hospital has been named as one of the Top 100 Hospitals in the United States for 2009, 2011, and 2012.

He is a Fellow of the American College of Healthcare Executives (ACHE), a member of many community boards, and an elder in the First Presbyterian Church. He is the past Chairman of the Michigan Health and Hospital Association Small and Rural Council.

MacLeod was honored with the Cadillac Citizen-of-the-Year award in 2004 and the American Hospital Association Grassroots Champion Award in 2012.

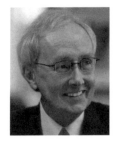

PHILIP H. MCCORKLE, JR.
President and CEO, Saint Mary's Health Care

CEO EXPERIENCE

4/2000–Present	Saint Mary's Health Care	Grand Rapids, MI
1/1997–7/1999	DeVos Children's Hospital	Grand Rapids, MI
1/1993–7/1999	Butterworth Hospital	Grand Rapids, MI

EDUCATION

Master of Healthcare Administration
The George Washington University, Washington, DC

B.S. Biology
Wake Forest University, Winston-Salem, NC

BACKGROUND

Since April 2000, McCorkle has served as President and CEO of Saint Mary's Health Care, a $450-million enterprise consisting of an acute care hospital, Advantage Health Physician Network (now Advantage Health/Saint Mary's Medical Group), three health clubs, five outreach health centers, The Lacks Cancer Center, Saint Mary's Southwest, and the Hauenstein Center. Under his direction and leadership, Saint Mary's has built and opened The Lacks Cancer Center and Saint Mary's Southwest, a comprehensive ambulatory care facility that is a joint venture with several physician groups. He also spearheaded the development of the Hauenstein Center, a comprehensive neuroscience center. A leader in the Grand Rapids community in fundraising, he has raised nearly $70 million in philanthropy since his appointment as CEO.

He is a Fellow of the American College of Healthcare Executives (ACHE) and a member of the Alliance for Health Board of Directors. He has also served as Chair of the Hospice of Michigan board. He was the first designated West Michigan Regional Market Executive for Trinity Health, a position he held from July 2006 through June 2010.

Prior to his appointment as President and CEO of Saint Mary's, he served as Executive Vice President of Spectrum Health and CEO of its downtown campus. Prior to the merger of Blodgett and Butterworth hospitals that resulted in Spectrum Health, he served in several executive positions, culminating in CEO at Butterworth Hospital in Grand Rapids, MI. He began his career at Byerly Hospital in Hartsville, SC.

McCorkle is married and has two sons and two grandsons.

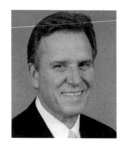

ROBERT MILEWSKI

Senior Vice President, Hospital Relations, Blue Cross
Blue Shield of Michigan

CEO EXPERIENCE

7/2006–11/2006	Mount Clemens Regional Medical Center	Mount Clemens, MI
9/1998–7/2006	Mount Clemens General Hospital	Mount Clemens, MI

EDUCATION

Master of Business Administration
Wayne State University, Detroit, MI

Master of Health Sciences
Wayne State University, Detroit, MI

B.S. Pharmacy
Wayne State University, Detroit, MI

BACKGROUND

Milewski is Senior Vice President and Special Assistant to the President for Hospital Relations for Blue Cross Blue Shield of Michigan. Since joining the Blues in 2007, he has held responsibilities for hospital and provider contracting, provider audit, claims processing, enrollment, billing, and customer service. He was president and CEO of Mount Clemens Regional Medical Center, which he had joined in 1993 as Executive Vice President and COO. Previously, he was Associate Hospital Director at William Beaumont Hospital in Royal Oak. From 1981 to 1987, he held various positions at Children's Hospital of Michigan in Detroit, including Director of Pharmacy, Assistant Administrator of Allied Health Services, and Associate Administrator of Operations.

He is a board member of the Alliance for Advancing Nonprofit Health Care, Center for Affordable Quality Healthcare (CAQH), SE Michigan Beacon Community, Citizens Research Council, and BCBSM Foundation.

He also is a Fellow and Past Regent of the American College of Healthcare Executives (ACHE) and Board Chairman of the Greater Detroit Area Health Council. He has also served as Chairman of the Midwest Healthcare Executives Group and Associates board, as well as a member of the Michigan Health and Hospital Association and the Leadership Macomb boards.

Milewski began his career as a staff pharmacist at William Beaumont Hospitals in Royal Oak and Troy.

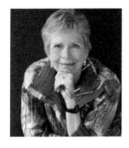

BETTY J. NOYES
President of Noyes & Associates Ltd.

CEO EXPERIENCE
7/1989–Present   Noyes and Associates Ltd.   Bainbridge Island, WA
1/1987–6/1989   Sierra Gateway Hospital   Clovis, CA

EDUCATION
Master of Public Health
Columbia University, New York, NY

Master of Nursing Administration
Teachers College of Columbia University, New York, NY

B.S. Nursing
State University of New York at Buffalo, Buffalo, NY

BACKGROUND
Noyes is President of Noyes & Associates Ltd., which she founded in 1989 and which offers management education courses, leadership assessment, and organization redesign and process improvement services. The emphasis of the company is the integration of mission with leadership performance and the belief that excellence in patient care and excellence in financial return are mutually interdependent.

Prior to establishing Noyes & Associates Ltd., she had developed 35 years of experience in healthcare administration across all phases of clinical and administrative management. Her administrative experience has been in multi-hospital systems, large university teaching facilities, and small for-profit hospitals in psychiatry and chemical dependency.

She has authored more than 18 articles and is frequently sought as a public speaker. She is an active member of various healthcare organizations nationwide.

Noyes was born in New York City and is part of a family of 13 registered nurses. She and her husband live on Bainbridge Island, WA.

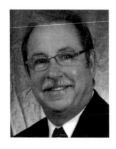

RICK O'CONNELL
Executive Vice President and COO, Hospital Networks for Trinity Health

CEO EXPERIENCE

5/1999–2/2008	Penrose St. Francis Health Services	Colorado Springs, CO
4/1995–4/1999	Lucerne Medical Center	Orlando, FL
1/1992–3/1993	Pembroke Pines Hospital	Pembroke Pines, FL

EDUCATION

B.B.A. Business Administration
Central State University, Edmond, OK

B.S. Hospital Administration
Oklahoma Baptist University, Shawnee, OK

BACKGROUND

As Executive Vice President and COO of Hospital Networks, O'Connell provides executive leadership and direction in the operations of all ministry organizations to ensure safe, high-quality healthcare delivery and services that meet the needs of each community. He focuses on building trust and strong relationships with boards, physicians, and associates of every level.

He recognizes and appreciates the diversity of challenges of each market Trinity Health serves. As healthcare enters a new age of reform, he is focusing his efforts on patient safety, growth initiatives, and improving performance.

Throughout his 37-year career, he has worked in operations with executive level management in both the corporate and hospital arena. His career experience includes President and CEO of the 522-bed Penrose-St. Francis Health Services in Colorado Springs. His other CEO positions have included Lucerne Medical Center in Orlando, Columbia Medical Center in Daytona Beach, and Pembroke Pines Hospital in Florida. He also served as COO/CFO of the Miami Heart Institute, the Miami Beach Community Hospital, and Doctors Hospital in Tulsa.

O'Connell is a champion of community involvement, having sat on many local boards. His efforts were recognized in 2004 when he was named Business Citizen of the Year by the Colorado Springs Chamber of Commerce.

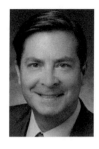

DAVID A. OLSON
Chief Strategy Officer and Senior Vice President,
Froedtert Health System

CEO EXPERIENCE

1/2012–9/2012	Froedtert Health–St. Joseph's Hospital	West Bend, WI
1/2010–10/2011	Columbia St. Mary's	Milwaukee, WI
5/1999–12/2009	Bay Area Medical Center	Marinette, WI

EDUCATION

Master of Business Administration
University of Iowa, Iowa City, IA

Master of Health Administration
University of Iowa, Iowa City, IA

B.S. Business Administration
University of Wisconsin–Eau Claire, Eau Claire, WI

BACKGROUND

In 2011, Olson was named Chief Strategy Officer and Senior Vice President for Froedtert Health System. He also served as President of Froedtert Health St. Joseph's Hospital. In 2010, Olson joined Columbia St. Mary's as President of their Ozaukee Hospital and an Executive Vice President of the system. For the prior 11 years, Olson was President and CEO of Bay Area Medical Center (BAMC), a 99-bed licensed acute care facility in Marinette, WI. He joined BAMC as COO in 1998, and was named President and CEO in 1999.

He served as President and CEO of Victory Medical Center in Stanley, WI, from 1994 to 1995, where he led the transition of the organization to Ministry Health Care. From 1994 to 1998, he served as Vice President of Administrative Services for St. Joseph's Hospital in Marshfield, WI, the flagship hospital of the Ministry Health Care System. He was also President of the Foundation of St. Joseph's Hospital. From 1986 to 1993, he rose through the administrative ranks to Vice President of Rehabilitation and Support Services at St. Luke's Hospital in Cedar Rapids, IA.

He is a Fellow of the American College of Healthcare Executives (ACHE). In 2001, he was selected as the organization's Hudgens Memorial Award winner for National Young Healthcare Executive of the Year. During 2010, Olson served as Chair of Wisconsin Hospital Association and currently serves as the Immediate Past Chair.

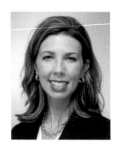

CARRIE OWEN PLIETZ

CEO, Sutter Medical Center

CEO EXPERIENCE
9/2011–Present   Sutter Medical Center   Sacramento, CA

EDUCATION
Master of Health Services Administration
Virginia Commonwealth University, Richmond, VA

B.S. Health Services Administration
James Madison University, Harrisonburg, VA

BACKGROUND
Owen Plietz was appointed CEO of Sutter Medical Center, Sacramento, in September 2011, and joined the center as COO in January 2011 after serving as COO at Mills-Peninsula Health Services, another Sutter Health affiliate. Sutter Medical Center, Sacramento, is a large tertiary medical center serving 29 counties composed of 823 beds, 3,600 employees, and 970 active medical staff.

She joined Mills-Peninsula Health Services as COO in 2008 after 9 years at Sutter Health's California Pacific Medical Center (CPMC). At Mills-Peninsula, she implemented Sutter Health's first acute care electronic health record and was a key driver in the journey to open its new $620 million medical center in Burlingame and $20 million new behavioral health center. She also spearheaded a major "patient affordability" initiative that helped drive down costs and created a successful approach to improving patient satisfaction that brings together caregivers each week to listen to the "Voice of the Patient" through satisfaction survey results, letters, and family comments.

She was most recently honored as one of *Modern Healthcare* magazine's Up and Comers 2011, and the 2010 Robert S. Hudgens Young Health Care Executive of the Year by the American College of Healthcare Executives (ACHE). She serves as Regent for ACHE Northern and Central California and ACHE Chapter Committee Member as well as sits on the Board for March of Dimes Greater Sacramento Division. She is past President of the California Association of Healthcare Leaders and past Chair of the ACHE Early Careerist Committee.

Owen Plietz lives in El Dorado Hills with her husband and two children.

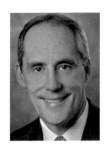

THOMAS M. PRISELAC
President and CEO, Cedars-Sinai Health System

CEO EXPERIENCE
1/1994–Present   Cedars-Sinai Health System   Los Angeles, CA

EDUCATION
Master of Health Services Administration
University of Pittsburgh, Pittsburgh, PA

B.S. Biology
Washington and Jefferson College, Washington, PA

BACKGROUND
Priselac is President and CEO of the Cedars-Sinai Health System, a position he has held since January 1994.

He has been associated with Cedars-Sinai since 1979. Prior to being named President and CEO, he was Executive Vice President from 1988 to 1993. Before joining Cedars-Sinai, he was on the executive staff of Montefiore Hospital in Pittsburgh, PA.

He has served the healthcare field in various roles during his career at Cedars-Sinai. He is a past Chair of the American Hospital Association Board of Trustees and also a past Chair of the Association of American Medical Colleges. Prior to those roles, he chaired the Hospital Association of Southern California, the California Healthcare Association, and the Association of American Medical Colleges Council of Teaching Hospitals.

The holder of the Warschaw/Law Endowed Chair in Healthcare Leadership at Cedars-Sinai Medical Center, Priselac also serves as an adjunct professor at the UCLA School of Public Health.

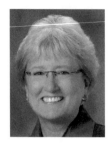

NANCY M. SCHLICHTING
CEO, Henry Ford Health System

CEO EXPERIENCE
6/2003–Present	Henry Ford Health System	Detroit, MI
8/2001–6/2003	Henry Ford Hospital	Detroit, MI
1/1994–1/1996	Riverside Methodist Hospitals	Columbus, OH

EDUCATION
Master of Business Administration, Hospital Administration, and Accounting
Cornell University, Ithaca, NY

A.B. Public Policy
Duke University, Durham, NC

BACKGROUND
Schlichting is CEO of Henry Ford Health System (HFHS), a nationally recognized $4.2 billion healthcare organization with 24,000 employees. She is credited with leading the health system through a dramatic financial turnaround and for achieving award-winning patient safety, customer service, and diversity initiatives. HFHS is the recipient of the 2011 Malcolm Baldrige National Quality Award. She joined HFHS in 1998 as its Senior Vice President and COO and was named President and CEO in 2003. Her career in healthcare administration spans 30 years of experience in senior-level executive positions.

She serves on many national and community boards: The Kresge Foundation; Walgreen Company; Federal Reserve Bank of Chicago–Detroit Branch; Detroit Regional Chamber (Chair); Citizen's Research Council of Michigan; Detroit Economic Club; and Downtown Detroit Partnership. She is also a member of the American College of Healthcare Executives (ACHE) and the Michigan Women's Forum.

Her most recent awards include *Becker's Hospital Review's* 50 Most Powerful People to Know in Healthcare and Women to Know in Health Care; *Modern Healthcare* magazine's 100 Most Powerful People in Healthcare and Top 25 Women in Healthcare (for a second time); Harvard Business School Club of Michigan Business Leader of the Year; Ernst & Young Spirit of Entrepreneurship Award; *Crain's Detroit Business's* Women to Watch; WJR's Women Who Lead; Crime Stoppers' Eleanor Josaitis Visionary Leader; Vanguard Community Development's E. L. Vann Visionary; Detroit's *Ambassador* magazine's Power Player; and *Health Care Weekly Review's* Health Care Executive of the Year.

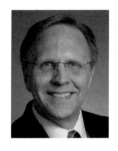

MICHAEL A. SLUBOWSKI

President and CEO, Sisters of
Charity of Leavenworth Health System

CEO EXPERIENCE

2/2012–Present	Sisters of Charity of Leavenworth Health System	Denver, CO
12/1994–3/1997	Providence Hospital and Medical Centers	Southfield, MI
1/1988–11/1990	Samaritan Physicians Center	Phoenix, AZ

EDUCATION

Master of Business Administration
Wayne State University, Detroit, MI

B.S. Business Administration
Wayne State University. Detroit, MI

BACKGROUND

Mike Slubowski began his career in hospital management more than 35 years ago and currently serves as President and CEO of Sisters of Charity of Leavenworth Health System (SCLHS). He provides executive leadership to SCLHS' 11 acute care facilities and numerous ambulatory facilities in California, Colorado, Montana, and Kansas. SCLHS has 15,000 FTE associates and $2.7 billion in annual net revenue.

He previously served as President of Health Networks for Trinity Health, the fourth-largest Catholic Health system in the U.S. He was responsible for Trinity Health's non-inpatient services and strategies, including ambulatory programs, physician practices, senior living communities, and home health services. He was also responsible for strategy and implementation of market-based Accountable Health Networks and Patient-Centered Medical Homes. Previous to that, he provided executive leadership to Trinity Health's Ministry Organizations (MOs) nationally, including hospitals and other health services.

He holds fellowships in both the American College of Healthcare Executives (ACHE), and the American College of Medical Practice Executives. He also serves in a variety of regional and national healthcare professional organizations, and is the past ACHE Regent for Eastern Michigan.

Slubowski is married and has twin adult daughters.

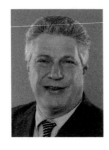

DAVID A. SPIVEY

President and CEO, St. Mary Mercy Hospital

CEO EXPERIENCE

| 6/2000–Present | St. Mary Mercy Hospital | Livonia, MI |
| 1/1998–6/2000 | Mercy Hospital Detroit | Detroit, MI |

EDUCATION

Master of Health Services Administration
University of Michigan, Ann Arbor, MI

Master of Business Administration
University of Michigan, Ann Arbor, MI

Bachelor of Arts
University of Michigan, Ann Arbor, MI

BACKGROUND

David Spivey has served as President and CEO of St. Mary Mercy Hospital for 11 years, and has worked with Trinity Health in a variety of management roles for 24 years. In addition to his leadership role at St. Mary Mercy Hospital, he chairs the Trinity Health system-wide Supply Chain Committee and is a member of its IT Executive Steering Team and Revenue Cycle Management Steering Committee. He also provides administrative oversight to Trinity's Mercy Primary Care Center, which provides uncompensated care to the uninsured on the east side of Detroit.

Under his leadership, St. Mary Mercy Hospital has won numerous awards, including HealthGrades Distinguished Hospital Award for Clinical Excellence 8 years in a row, and Thomson Reuters Top 100 Hospital Award 2 years in a row. In 2010, he oversaw the implementation of the hospital's Graduate Medical Education program, which has grown to more than 130 residents and 7 programs.

David Spivey is actively involved in numerous community activities, including the Board of the Livonia Chamber of Commerce, Member of the Rotary Club of Livonia, and past President and Board Member of the University of Michigan School of Public Health, Health Management, and Policy Alumni Association. He also serves on the Regional Blood Services Board of the American Red Cross Southeastern Michigan Blood Region.

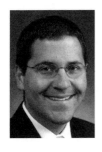

DAVID A. STARK

President and CEO, Blank Children's Hospital
Executive Vice President, Iowa Health–Des Moines

CEO EXPERIENCE

8/2009–Present	Blank Children's Hospital	Des Moines, IA
2/2009–8/2009	Advocate Lutheran General Hospital	Park Ridge, IL

EDUCATION

Master of Hospital Administration
University of Iowa, Iowa City, IA

B.S. in Management
Iowa State University, Ames, IA

BACKGROUND

Stark serves as President and COO of Blank Children's Hospital and Executive Vice President of Iowa Health–Des Moines. He joined the Iowa Health–Des Moines System in 1996 and has served as Executive Vice President and COO for Iowa Methodist Medical Center and Iowa Lutheran Hospital.

He is a Fellow in the American College of Healthcare Executives (ACHE) and received the 2008 national Robert S. Hudgens Memorial Award for a Young Healthcare Executive. He is a 2000 graduate of the Greater Des Moines Leadership Institute, Member of Iowa State University College of Business Management and Marketing Council, Member of Iowa Hospital Association, Member of Iowa Regents Advisory council, and a Member of Rotary. He serves on the boards of First American Bank, Iowa Public Television, Blank Park Zoo, and the YMCA.

Stark resides in Johnston, IA, with his wife and their four children.

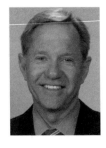

QUINT STUDER
Founder & Board Chairman, Studer Group

CEO EXPERIENCE
1/2000–9/2011   Studer Group   Gulf Breeze, FL
6/1996–1/2000   Baptist Hospital   Pensacola, FL

EDUCATION
Master of Science in Education
University of Wisconsin–Whitewater, Whitewater, WI

B.A. Education
University of Wisconsin–Whitewater, Whitewater, WI

BACKGROUND
Studer spent 10 years as a teacher before entering the healthcare industry in 1984 as a Community Relations Representative. From then until he founded Studer Group in 2000, he served as Department Director, Vice President, and Senior Vice President at a number of organizations, as well as President of Baptist Hospital in Pensacola, FL.

A recipient of the 2010 Malcolm Baldrige National Quality Award, Studer Group implements evidence-based leadership systems that help clients attain and sustain outstanding results in more than 800 hospitals and organizations across the U.S. Together they serve a "national learning lab" in which best practices are harvested, tested, refined, and shared with all healthcare organizations through peer-reviewed journal articles, Studer Group publications, and products designed to accelerate change. For the fifth year in a row, Studer Group was named one of the 2012 Best Small & Medium Workplaces by Great Places to Work®, ranking fourth in the nation.

He is a *Wall Street Journal* best-selling author and has written six books. His latest, *The Great Employee Handbook*, is geared toward employees at all levels, and the insightful tips he shares are not what you will find in any training manual.

Studer remains in the field developing tools and techniques designed to make organizations better. He has been called a "fire starter" for igniting the flame in each of us to be the best that we can be and to always connect back to purpose.

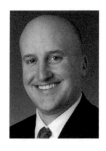

KEVIN L. UNGER
President and CEO, Poudre Valley Hospital

CEO EXPERIENCE
11/2006–Present   Poudre Valley Hospital   Fort Collins, CO

EDUCATION
Master of Health Services Administration
University of Colorado, Denver, CO

B.A. Sociology
Colorado State University, Fort Collins,CO

BACKGROUND
Unger came to Poudre Valley Health System in 2001 and has held the positions of Vice President of Planning and Strategic Development and Vice President of Operations for Poudre Valley Hospital. In 2005 he was named the President and CEO of Poudre Valley Hospital.

Before joining Poudre Valley Hospital, he held positions at University Hospital and the University of Colorado Health Sciences Center in Denver. He also spent 2 years as a healthcare consultant with First Consulting Group headquartered in Long Beach, CA.

In 2009, he received the Robert S. Hudgens Young Healthcare Executive of the Year award through the American College of Healthcare Executives (ACHE). In 2007, Modern Healthcare magazine recognized him as an "up and comer," designating him as one of the 12 young "rising stars" of the healthcare administration profession in the country. In 2002, he was named as one of northern Colorado's "40 under 40" by the Northern Colorado Business Report as an individual who has had an impact on his or her organization, has made significant contributions of time and talent to the community, and has shown potential for being a leader as the 21st century progresses.

A native of Fort Collins, CO, Unger is currently completing a doctor of philosophy in organizational development and change at Colorado State University. He and his wife are the proud parents of three children.

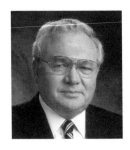

GAIL L. WARDEN
President Emeritus, Henry Ford Health System

CEO EXPERIENCE

6/1988–12/2003	Henry Ford Health System	Detroit, MI
1/1981–12/1987	Group Health Cooperative	Seattle, WA

EDUCATION

Honorary Doctorate in Public Administration
Rosalind Franklin University of Medicine and Science, North Chicago, IL

Master of Hospital Administration
University of Michigan, Ann Arbor, MI

A.B. Liberal Arts
Dartmouth College, Hanover, NH

BACKGROUND

Warden serves as President Emeritus of Detroit-based Henry Ford Health System and served as its President and CEO from 1988–2003. He is also Professor of Health Management and Policy at the University of Michigan, School of Public Health.

He is an elected member of the Institute of Medicine of the National Academy of Sciences. He served on its Board of Health Care Services, Committee on Quality Health Care in America; chaired the Committee on the Future of Emergency Medicine in the United States; and served two terms on its Governing Council. He is Chairman Emeritus of the National Quality Forum, Chairman Emeritus of the National Committee for Quality Assurance, a past Chairman of the American Hospital Association, and the Chair Emeritus of National Center for Healthcare Leadership. He is an Emeritus member of the Robert Wood Johnson Foundation Board of Trustees and serves on the RAND Health Board of Advisors.

Warden holds the position of Vice Chairman and Trustee for the Rosalind Franklin University of Medicine and Science's Board of Directors, and he chairs the Detroit Wayne County Health Authority and the Detroit Zoological Society. He is also a Director for the National Research Corporation's Board of Directors in Lincoln, NE, and the Picker Institute. He served as a Director of Comerica, Inc., from 1990–2006.

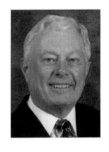

DONALD C. WEGMILLER

Chairman and CEO, C-Suite Resources
Chairman and CEO, Scottsdale Institute

CEO EXPERIENCE

4/1993–4/2004	INTEGRATED Healthcare Strategies	Minneapolis, MN
11/1976–4/1993	Allina Health System	Minneapolis, MN
10/1966–10/1976	Fairview Southdale Hospital	Minneapolis, MN

EDUCATION

Master of Health Services Administration
University of Minnesota, Minneapolis, MN

B.A. Business Economics and Psychology
University of Minnesota, Minneapolis, MD

BACKGROUND

Wegmiller is Chairman and CEO of C-Suite Resources, a business intelligence advisory firm specializing in providing market intelligence on the healthcare industry firms serving hospitals and health systems. He also serves as Chairman Emeritus of INTEGRATED Healthcare Strategies, the nation's leading authority on executive compensation and physician compensation for healthcare organizations. He previously served as the firm's Chairman and CEO.

He also serves as Chairman and CEO of Scottsdale Institute. Founded 16 year ago, the institute serves the healthcare sector through its focus on collaborative efforts in information technology.

He continues to hold policy positions in state and national healthcare associations. He has served on the boards of numerous publicly held corporations over the past 20 years, and currently serves on the boards of three public companies, two private companies, and two company advisory boards.

From 1986 to 1988, Wegmiller served as a chairman officer of the American Hospital Association, serving in 1987 as the organization's chairman, the highest-elected office. He was also named a Fellow in the American College of Healthcare Executives (ACHE), and in August 2002 was named by *Modern Healthcare* magazine as one of healthcare's 100 Most Powerful People.

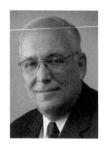

JACK WEINER
President and CEO,
St. Joseph Mercy Oakland

CEO EXPERIENCE

12/2003–Present	St. Joseph Mercy Hospital Oakland	Pontiac, MI
5/1998–12/2003	St. Joseph's Mercy Macomb	Clinton Township, MI
5/1992–12/1995	Northeastern Hospital of Philadelphia	Philadelphia, PA
1/1989–5/1992	Cuyahoga Falls General Hospital	Cuyahoga Falls, OH
1/1986–1/1989	Mount Clemens General Hospital	Mount Clemens, MI

EDUCATION

Master of Health Services Administration
University of Michigan, Ann Arbor, MI

Doctor of Clinical Pharmacy
Wayne State University, Detroit, MI

B.S. Pharmacy
University of Buffalo, Buffalo, NY

BACKGROUND

As President and CEO of St. Joseph Mercy Oakland (SJMO), Weiner has led the organization in a major cultural transformation and a $300 million campus redevelopment, which includes construction of a new Patient Tower that will include state-of-the-art technology found in only one other hospital in the country. Under his leadership, SJMO became the regional leader in clinical quality and safety. Previous redevelopment includes: a new surgical pavilion; the Robert Gustafson Wing (housing a new emergency center, an imaging center and pharmacy, and a three-floor patient tower with 90 private rooms); and implementation of the patient Electronic Medical Record (EMR) system, which expands throughout southeastern Michigan Trinity Hospitals and physician offices. SJMO's Michigan Stroke Network has led an initiative that improves the care of stroke patients in hospitals throughout Michigan.

Prior to joining SJMO in 2003, he served as President and CEO of St. Joseph Mercy Macomb, where, under his leadership, an open-heart surgery program and $30 million expansion program were launched. He began his administrative career as an administrative resident at Oakwood Hospital in Dearborn, MI.

Weiner resides in Birmingham, Michigan, with his wife Faye.

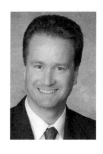

SEAN WILLIAMS
President and CEO, Mercy Medical Center

CEO EXPERIENCE

3/2010–Present	Mercy Medical Center	Clinton, IA
10/2004–3/2010	Jones Regional Medical Center	Anamosa, IA

EDUCATION

Master of Healthcare Administration
Des Moines University, Des Moines, IA

B.A. Economics
Loras College, Dubuque, IA

BACKGROUND

Williams is President and CEO of Mercy Medical Center in Clinton, Iowa.

Williams is a Fellow in the American College of Healthcare Executives (ACHE). He has taught at the graduate level and has been recognized by his peers with the ACHE Early Career Executive Award for Iowa, and was named to a regional "40 under 40" list of up-and-coming executives. He was recently awarded the Iowa Hospital Association Young Executive Achievement Award for 2012.

Index

Note: *f* indicates figures, *t* indicates tables.